Flexible Working and Training for Doctors and Dentists

A practical guide

Edited by

Anne Hastie

Director of Postgraduate General Practice Education
London Deanery

Foreword by

Elisabeth Paice

Dean Director of Postgraduate Medical and Dental Education
London Deanery

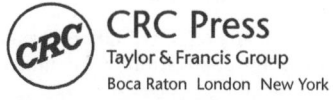
CRC Press
Taylor & Francis Group
Boca Raton London New York

CRC Press is an imprint of the
Taylor & Francis Group, an **informa** business

First published 2006 by Radcliffe Publishing

Published 2018 by CRC Press
Taylor & Francis Group
6000 Broken Sound Parkway NW, Suite 300
Boca Raton, FL 33487-2742

© 2006 by Ann Hastie
CRC Press is an imprint of Taylor & Francis Group, an Informa business

No claim to original U.S. Government works

ISBN-13: 978-1-84619-025-4 (pbk)

Visit the Taylor & Francis Web site at
http://www.taylorandfrancis.com

and the CRC Press Web site at
http://www.crcpress.com

Anne Hastie has asserted her right under the Copyright, Designs and Patents Act, 1998, to be identified as editor of this work.

The editor and publisher do not accept any responsibility or legal liability for any errors in the text or for the misuse or misapplication of any material in this text.

British Library Cataloguing in Publication Data

A catalogue record for this book is available from the British Library.

Typeset by Ann Buchan (Typesetters), Middlesex

Contents

Foreword

Anne Hastie has pulled together the first book I can recall seeing on flexible training and working in medicine and dentistry. The subject matter is highly topical. The proportion of women in medicine and dentistry rises each year, and with it the demand for less-than-full-time working.

The flexible training scheme was a brilliant concept when it was first introduced in the 1970s. I was an early beneficiary of the scheme, which provided me with the opportunity to train part-time for seven years while I produced and raised three children. Naturally enough, I have been a staunch champion of flexible training ever since. So it may come as a shock if I say that I would now like to see the flexible training scheme disappear. The reason is that that what was once a very unusual career pathway is becoming better and better travelled. It is time that training flexibly came to be seen as just another training option, and not a special scheme. It is time that flexible training joined the mainstream of training. The recent pay agreement, which ensures that salaries reflect working hours, is already proving helpful in achieving this. So is a general move away from the 'supernumerary' post to a slot share or reduced sessions in a full-time post. The more flexible training is regarded as ordinary, the less flexible trainees will have to struggle to get the experience and training they need. Competency-based curricula should ensure that all trainees progress according to the skills they acquire, not the hours served. There is a way to go before that becomes a reality. In the meantime, hundreds of trainees in each region of the country, and in each specialty, are enjoying the reduced hours and greater personal time afforded by the flexible training scheme or by the range of options available to doctors and dentists with well-founded reasons for wishing to work less than full-time.

This book explores the rules and regulations around the flexible training scheme as it currently functions, as well as exploring a range of other options for non-standardised career pathways, whether in primary or secondary care, medicine or dentistry. There are also chapters on flexible training and working for doctors and dentists with aspirations to become academics, managers or medical educationalists. The glass ceiling has long been breached, and working less than full-time is no barrier to success in a wide variety of areas. This book will prove a useful resource for any doctors or dentists who are contemplating working less than full-time themselves, or who guide or manage others making these choices. Clinical tutors, course organisers and deanery staff will find it invaluable and unique.

Professor Elisabeth Paice
Dean Director
London Deanery
July 2006

About the editor

Anne Hastie is currently Director of Postgraduate General Practice Education in the London Deanery. She qualified from St George's Hospital Medical School in 1974 and, following her GP training, was a full-time GP in south London before joining the London Deanery in 2001. She was a trainer for 15 years, a GP tutor for 10 years and a course organiser for the GP retainer scheme for eight years. Dr Hastie has a long-standing interest in career advice and flexible training and working. This began because she did not have the opportunity to work part-time while her children were young and she did not want other GPs to have the same lack of choice. Her research interests are in medical education and she has published papers on the GP retainer scheme, the flexible career scheme, the GP returner scheme and on prolonged study leave. She writes regularly for the *British Medical Journal* Career Advice Zone.

Dr Hastie obtained an MSc with distinction in health sciences at St George's in 2000 and, in the same year, was awarded an MBE for services to medicine.

List of contributors

Antony Americano

Antony Americano is Head of Human Resources and Central Services at the London Deanery, University of London. He is a Fellow of the Chartered Institute of Personnel and Development and has a Masters degree in organisational behaviour from Birkbeck College, University of London. He has also published on management and general equalities issues.

Induja Bandara

Dr Bandara has been a GP for 10 years and is an undergraduate teacher at Guy's, King's and St Thomas' Medical School. She has been a programme director for higher professional education in the south-east and south-west London sectors since 2002. Dr Bandara has a particular interest in the work and education of salaried and sessional GPs, having published research and articles in these areas. She represents salaried and sessional GPs for the Lambeth Local Medical Council. She has an MSc in general practice and is currently studying for an MA in academic practice.

Nav Chana

Nav Chana is a GP principal in Mitcham, Surrey, and is an associate director for the London Deanery. He has been a trainer and a course organiser. For the past 10 years he has been an examiner for the MRCGP, and is currently involved in developing workplace-based assessment for the Royal College of General Practitioners. Dr Chana is a member of the executive board of the National Association of Primary Care and his special interests include transforming chronic care and primary care workforce development. He is also Chair of the Primary Care Workforce Development Steering Group of South West London Strategic Health Authority.

Clare Etherington

Dr Clare Etherington qualified at University College Hospital Medical School, London, in 1986. She is a full-time GP in Harrow and a GP trainer on the Northwick Park Vocational Training Scheme. She is currently an educational supervisor to a flexible career scheme, doctor and trainer for a doctor on an innovative training post (shared general practice and hospital post). Dr Etherington has been involved in mentoring on both the North Thames Non-principals Mentoring Project and the Hillingdon Mentoring Scheme. She is one of the programme directors for higher professional education (education for GPs within the first two years of qualifying) in the London Deanery and her area is North West Thames.

Beverley Gainey

Beverley Gainey read business studies and worked at ICI before following a management training programme with the Inland Revenue. She qualified as an accountant with the National Audit Office, and after gaining an MBA at Cranfield, she joined an NHS Regional Health Authority where she developed an interest in education and training finance. Beverley is currently the Head of Educational Resource Development at the London Deanery and part of her role is to oversee the administration of flexible training for all hospital medical and dental training grades in London. In addition she also overseas the administration of specialist registrars in Essex, Hertfordshire, Kent, Surrey and Sussex.

Ann Griffin

Ann Griffin is a sessional GP working in north London. She is involved in postgraduate education as a programme director for higher professional education at the London Deanery and in undergraduate teaching as a clinical teaching fellow at the Royal Free and University College London Medical School. She passed MRCGP in 2001 and was given a distinguished teachers award from University College London in 2003. She has just submitted her masters in medical education degree thesis on evaluating clinical teaching in primary care.

Imtiaz Gulamali

Imtiaz Gulamali has a broad range of experience in primary and secondary care as well as general practice education. He has worked as a hospital practitioner and also as the lead for diabetes in a primary care trust. He worked as a GP tutor for five years and is currently a trainer, course organiser and associate director of postgraduate general practice education in the London Deanery.

Ian Hastie

Dr Hastie is Dean for Postgraduate Medicine, London and the national lead postgraduate dean for several specialties. He is a consultant and senior lecturer in geriatric medicine at St George's Hospital and Medical School and is also President of the geriatric medicine section of the European Union of Medical Specialties, a member of the specialist advisory committee for geriatric medicine and member of the national training committee of the British Geriatrics Society.

Elizabeth Jones

Elizabeth Jones qualified as a dentist, with honours, from Birmingham University in 1977 (Gold Medal winner). She initially worked in general dental practice but then entered specialist training in orthodontics at the Royal Dental

Hospital, London, and Kingston Hospital. Following this she became a part-time (flexible) senior registrar at Guy's and St George's. She has worked as a part-time consultant at West Middlesex University Hospital and the Chelsea and Westminster Hospital, treating patients with cleft lip and palate, and currently works at Kingston Hospital and Ashford Hospital. Dr Jones joined the London Deanery as an associate dean for secondary care dentistry in 2001 and became the Dean for Postgraduate Dentistry in 2003. She is the national lead dean for orthodontics and has served as an elected member of the special advisory committee for orthodontics. She has a certificate in teaching and is an examiner for the Membership in Orthodontics (for both the intercollegiate examination and the Royal College of Surgeons of England).

Neil Jackson

Neil Jackson first entered general practice in 1974 (he retired from active medical clinical practice in 1999 after 25 years as a full-time principal) and quickly developed an interest in education and training. He is a former GP trainer, course organiser and associate regional adviser in general practice. He is now Postgraduate Dean for General Practice in the London Deanery and Honorary Professor of Medical Education at Queen Mary College (Barts and the Royal London Hospitals). He is a former MRCGP examiner and the author of various books, book chapters, peer-referenced papers and articles on general practice/primary care/education and training issues. For the past few years he has worked as a visiting family medicine and primary care consultant in countries of the former Russian Federation, including Georgia and Uzbekistan, and, more recently, in Japan and Poland.

Leanda Kroll

Dr Leanda Kroll is a senior lecturer in medical education (part-time) at St George's, University of London, with special responsibility for students' welfare and academic progression. Previously she held a flexible job in academic medicine at St George's, one of five five-year flexible posts available at London medical schools under the Chadburn lectureship scheme. She has written about this experience for BMJ Careers. She originally trained flexibly as a specialist registrar in child and adolescent psychiatry, but a research interest in how doctors can help families to discuss a parent's cancer diagnosis, led her into medical education, after gaining her certificate of completion of specialist training (CCST).

Susan La Brooy

Susan La Brooy is an associate dean with the London Deanery and is responsible for the flexible careers scheme for hospitals. She is a geriatrician and medical director at the Hillingdon Hospital, an acute district general hospital in west London. Throughout her career, she has been involved in service development, innovation and improvement at both local and national levels. Her interest in training and education led her to work first as chair of a specialty training committee in the London Deanery and then as an associate dean.

Elisabeth Paice

Professor Elisabeth Paice is Dean Director of Postgraduate Medical and Dental Education for London. This role involves commissioning, managing and quality assuring postgraduate training for over 8000 doctors and dentists in London and the surrounding area. She was previously consultant rheumatologist at Whittington Hospital, where she also was Clinical Tutor (1990–1993). She became an associate dean for North Thames East in 1993, with special responsibility for pre-registration house officers, senior house officers and flexible training. From 1995 to 2001 she was Dean Director of Postgraduate Medical and Dental Education for North Thames. Professor Paice was overseas expert on the Australian Medical Council team accrediting the Royal Australasian College of Physicians in 2004. She has published on the European Working Time Directive (EWTD) and the hospital at night; stress and disillusionment in doctors; the relationship between trainers and trainees; appraisal and the management of performance; identifying doctors in difficulty; workplace bullying; women in medicine; and other aspects of medical careers and postgraduate medical training.

Hazel Richardson

Hazel Richardson has been an inner-city GP for the last 30 years. She has a strong interest in education, having been a trainer for many years and, more recently, a higher professional education programme director. Her four children were brought up in an era when there were very few flexible career opportunities so she recognises the difficulties of combining a career with childcare and welcomes new developments in flexible training.

Jane Roberts

Jane H Roberts is an undergraduate clinical lecturer (part-time) at Durham in Phase 1 Medicine where she is the academic lead for personal and professional development. She is also a salaried GP with a special interest in substance misuse on which she has written for BMJ Careers and the *British Journal of General Practice*. Dr Roberts' research interests lie in understanding the obstacles to encouraging cultural competence in medical undergraduates and developing effective educational material to improve cultural responsiveness in healthcare settings. She sits on the BMA Medical Academic Staff committee and is keen to contribute to a change in the present culture of medical academia, which could lead to healthier working lives for all doctors in academia.

John Spicer

John Spicer has been a GP in south London for 20 years, and still is. He has a portfolio working week, including posts as an associate director of postgraduate general practice education for the London Deanery and as a clinical lecturer in medical law and ethics at St George's, University of London. He also teaches on a postgraduate certificate of education for primary care teachers. Sometimes he doesn't work at all.

Sally Smith

Sally Smith has been a GP principal for 13 years and has been involved in GP education for the last 10 years, as a GP tutor, trainer, higher professional education programme director and student tutor. Her involvement with new doctors has helped maintain her enthusiasm for general practice. Sally has completed a certificate in medical education (Dundee). She is an enthusiastic new recruit to the pleasures of learning to play tennis and also dances 'Ceroc' — a form of modern jive.

Tim Swanwick

Tim Swanwick is Director of Postgraduate General Practice in the London Deanery and an honorary senior lecturer at Imperial College, London. He has a broad interest in medical education and has taught and written extensively on many aspects of postgraduate education and training, including educational management and leadership. Recent publications include *The Management Handbook for Primary Care*, *The Study Guide for General Practice Training* and *The General Practice Journey*. Tim also continues in clinical general practice on the flexible careers scheme.

Rebecca Viney

Rebecca Viney is Associate Director of Postgraduate General Practice Education for sessional GPs at the London Deanery. In her time she has been a GP partner, GP retainer, locum and is currently a flexible career scheme GP. For the last nine years she has been involved with promoting continuing professional development opportunities for sessional GPs, both nationally and via the London Deanery. Dr Viney also works as a GP appraiser and in the past has been education lead on a preventive care group/primary care trust, a GP tutor and course organiser.

Introduction

Neil Jackson

One of the important features of modernising the National Health Service (NHS) is the development of its workforce to meet the needs of the communities it serves. The kind of workforce required must be fit for practice and purpose, with the ability to work in multi-professional/multi-disciplinary teams of healthcare professionals and capable of sustained learning and development. Quality service provision of healthcare for patients relies upon a highly trained and motivated NHS workforce, within which staff working on a flexible basis must find their place as a valuable workforce resource.

Approximately one million people work for the NHS, and we need to ensure that we plan and develop the NHS workforce by making the best use of the investment in it to provide the most effective care for patients. This fundamental principle was highlighted in *A Health Service of All the Talents: Developing the NHS Workforce.*[1] This report emphasised the key features of modernising the NHS workforce, that is:

- *Team working*, across professional and organisational boundaries.
- *Flexible working*, to make best use of the range of skills and knowledge possessed by staff.
- *Streamlined workforce planning and development*, which stems from the needs of patients not professionals.
- *Maximising the contribution of all staff to patient care*, doing away with professional barriers, which dictate that only nurses or doctors can provide particular kinds of care.
- *Modernising education and training*, to ensure that staff are equipped with the skills they need to work in a complex, changing NHS.
- *Developing new, more flexible careers*, for staff of all professions.
- *Expanding the workforce*, to meet future demands.

In summary, the report recommended a future health service of all the talents, and this would require a process of reform, including a change in the way staff work in the NHS, a key principle being flexible training, working and career development.

The importance of staff development and new working practices, including flexible working, was again highlighted in *The NHS Plan*,[2] which stated that 'NHS staff, at every level, are key to reform'. This document recognised the need for the NHS to better support and involve staff in improving care for patients through liberating the talent and skills of *all* the workforce, whether full-time or part-time.

In keeping with the process of reform, new principles underpinning the arrangements for flexible training have recently been published by the NHS.[3] These principles appreciate that less-than-full-time training should equate to full-time training when it comes to promoting a work–life balance, and include strategies such as caring for junior doctors' dependents, childcare provision and family-friendly work or training rotations. The number of doctors and dentists applying for flexible training is increasing each year as more women qualify, and many will wish to continue working on a less-than-full-time basis after qualification. This so-called 'feminisation' of the medical and dental workforce will affect future workforce planning and working practice. This, in turn, will need to be taken into account as we begin to implement the patient-led NHS,[4] the aims of which include strengthening commissioning in the NHS, achieving management cost savings and patient-centred service development. The latter will require effective workforce planning and the support of a skilled, flexible workforce.

Although the recruitment of healthcare professionals is crucial to the NHS as an employer in terms of adequate numbers and skill mixes across various professional groups, so, too, is the retention and development of staff. This applies to both the primary and secondary care sectors of the NHS and the employment of full-time and less-than-full-time doctors, dentists and professionals allied to medicine.

There are many principles which influence the retention and development of NHS staff. Some of these are employer- or employee-specific, and some are shared between employer and employee, as summarised below.[5]

Employer-specific principles

- Retaining and developing the right number of healthcare professionals with the right knowledge, skills and attitudes to deliver quality service provision for patients.
- Defining and implementing a value-based approach to challenge abusive and inappropriate behaviour in the workplace, such as prejudice, bullying and violence.
- Appropriate induction programmes for all new staff members.
- Planning staff development to underpin corporate and clinical governance.
- Having an appropriate performance management system within the employing organisation related to retention and development issues.

- Putting support systems in place to manage stress and to encourage reflection in daily working lives.
- Maintaining concern for all employees, at all levels, in the employing organisation; recognising and developing potential in each staff member and developing leadership qualities when appropriate.
- Securing sufficient resources to ensure investment in staff development.

Employee-specific principles

- Staff loyalty and commitment to the employing organisation and the NHS as a whole.
- Quality of working life for staff, particularly during 'out-of-hours' service provision.
- Regular appraisal and feedback on performance to encourage personal and professional development.
- 'Family-friendly' policies within the employing organisation to support flexible working for mothers with young children, and so on.
- Fair rates of pay for employees and incentive schemes where appropriate.

Shared principles

- Shared values, aims and objectives between employers and employees at all levels within the NHS employing organisation.
- Corporate responsibility for retaining and developing staff to include input at board level and throughout the organisation, including individual employees or employee representatives.
- Learning together across professional and disciplinary boundaries at organisational team and individual healthcare professional levels.
- Maintaining an appropriate balance between personal and professional development and employability in the NHS, that is, continuing professional development for healthcare professionals, which links personal and professional development needs to the wider needs of the employing organisation and the NHS as a whole.

As far as continuing professional development is concerned, a culture of lifelong learning and reflective practice must be encouraged for all doctors and dentists, whether full-time or less-than-full-time in the NHS. This will enable them to meet the challenge of a fast-changing world, medical and dental advances, new technologies and new approaches to patient care.

References

1   Secretary of State for Health (2000) *A Health Service of All the Talents: developing the NHS workforce*. Department of Health, London.

2 Secretary of State for Health (2000) *The NHS Plan: a plan for investment, a plan for reform.* Department of Health, London.

3 NHS Confederation (Employers) (2005) *Doctors in Flexible Training: principles underpinning the new arrangements for flexible training.* NHS Employers, Leeds.

4 Department of Health (2005) *Creating a Patient Led NHS: delivering the NHS improvement plan.* Department of Health, London.

5 Jackson N (2003) Work based learning and the retention and development of the NHS workforce. *Journal of Work Based Learning in Primary Care* **1**, 5–9.

CHAPTER 1

Setting the scene

Anne Hastie

Introduction

Medicine as a career has seen many changes in recent decades for a variety of reasons, some driven by the profession, others by government initiatives as well as external factors. The number of women working in medicine has increased every decade since the introduction of the National Health Service (NHS) in 1948, and it is predicted that women doctors will outnumber men by 2012.[1] Economic factors mean that many more women continue to work after becoming parents and the high divorce rate in the UK has not escaped the medical profession, placing a financial burden on both partners. Men and women are seeking a better work–life balance and the demand for part-time and flexible ways of training and working has been turned into an increasing reality. This has been supported and encouraged by the Department of Health through the 'Improving Working Lives' initiative.[2]

Historical background

Between 1950 and 1973 women were admitted to medical schools on a restricted-quota system. In 1973 the Sex Discrimination Act was introduced so the restricted quotas had to be abolished and by 1992 women had achieved parity in the numbers of medical school entrants. 1990 saw the hours of work for junior hospital doctors reduced to 72 hours a week and the European Working Time Directive[3] will reduce this further to 48 hours a week by 2009. However, these hours remain excessive for many women and some men.

Allen[4,5,6] extensively researched factors affecting women doctors, which attracted a lot of attention from the medical profession and the Department of Health. The research showed that in 1986 only 3% of women doctors (and no men) were in part-time training posts, although one-third were considering it in the future and there was a definite imbalance between supply and demand for part-time training. At the same time only 4% of women doctors were in part-time career posts, although 97% thought there should be greater availability, especially job-sharing opportunities. Allen's research indicated the need for a radical reassessment of the medical career structure and the way it was structured, with more opportunities for flexible training and working.

Davidson *et al.*[7] followed the career destinations of doctors who qualified in 1977 and Lambert and Goldacre[8] followed those who qualified in 1988. These workers showed that seven years after qualifying in 1988, 53% of women working in general practice and 20% working in hospital specialties worked part-time. Eighteen years after qualifying in 1977 the number of doctors working part-time in general practice was similar, at 51%, but the number of women working part-time in hospital specialties had risen to 42%.

There have been long-standing concerns about medical workforce planning, which is complex and has had a fragmented approach in the past,[9] and studies have highlighted the need for medical workforce planning to take into account the whole-time equivalent years of work. The number of women doctors shown not to be working is significantly less than in other professions,[10] but the high cost of training means it is worth trying to retain these doctors.

Current trends

Traditional patterns of work are no longer acceptable to many doctors in the medical profession who are looking for a better work–life balance: 48% of doctors (24% male and 74% female) who qualified in 1995 indicated that they might wish to work part-time at some point in their career[11] and one of the challenges will be making this a reality. Full-time work is still the norm and this retains a higher status in comparison to some part-time arrangements. However, working patterns are beginning to change, with increasing opportunities to work part-time. Although women are the main gender wanting to work flexibly there is an increasing demand from men, which may have helped contribute towards a greater acceptance of new working patterns.

The NHS Plan,[12] published in 2000, was closely followed by a consultation document, *A Health Service of all the Talents: Developing the NHS Workforce*,[9] which identified the need for investment and reform, and the Department of Health acknowledged the need for flexible working environments for doctors at various stages of their careers.[13] This became part of the consultation brief to develop the NHS workforce,[9] with an emphasis on flexible training and working in order to make the best use of the wide range of skills and knowledge available. In 2004 responsibility for employment issues and promoting the NHS as an employer was devolved to NHS Employers.

The Postgraduate Medical Education and Training Board (PMETB) took over the statutory responsibility for approving postgraduate medical education and training from the Specialist Training Authority (STA) and the Joint Committee on Postgraduate Training for General Practice (JCPTGP) on 30 September 2005.

New regulations will allow the PMETB to be more flexible in the type of training and experience that can be approved in order to allow doctors to be eligible to become consultants or GPs.

Career counselling

The importance of career counselling before choosing to enter medical training, and throughout undergraduate and postgraduate training, has been increasingly acknowledged, although many doctors still make career decisions by a process of elimination.[14] There is a need to develop career counselling, including tools appropriate to medicine. However, counselling also needs to be available throughout doctors' working careers and into retirement.

Modernising medical careers

In 2003 the Department of Health[15] first published details of modernising medical careers in response to a proposal from the Chief Medical Officer to review the house officer grade.[16] This modernisation has resulted in a reorganisation of postgraduate training for doctors, with the following main changes.

- The introduction of a two-year foundation programme to replace the Pre-registration House Officer (PRHO) and first Senior House Officer (SHO) years.
- The development of a 'run-through' grade for specialty training, including general practice.

A more flexible approach will be required to fit in with the European Working Time Directive and the demography of those entering medical school. There also needs to be the opportunity to change specialty training.

New contracts

New contracts are now in place for hospital consultants and general practitioners (GPs) after considerable negotiation between the profession and the Department of Health. The new 2003 consultant contract is the only contract available to new consultants, although some consultants already in post chose to stay on the previous contract. The new contract is based on a full-time week of 10 four-hour programmed activities, and doctors can choose to work part-time in consultation with their employing trust. Each consultant has a job plan, which is meant to take into account the full range of services they provide, including management and teaching.[17] It is hoped the new contract will allow more flexible working arrangements and improve part-time opportunities. Employers are able to offer annual contracts so consultants can vary the programmed activities they work each week to fit with personal commitments.

In 2004 there was also the introduction of a new contract for general practice,[18] which replaced the previous 1990 contract. GPs are now paid for essential (core) services and quality care for chronic disease. In addition, they can contract to provide enhanced services, which are negotiated locally. Enhanced services include the development of practitioners with special interest (PwSIs), which has enabled doctors who did significant amounts of training in another specialty and GPs who have developed additional skills to be paid for providing their expertise.

Practices receive a global sum, which represents practice income and not individual GPs' income as was the case under the 1990 contract. This enables practices to be more flexible in the way GPs are employed in their practice, for example as partners or salaried GPs. As a result there are increasing numbers of GPs working in salaried posts, many of whom are part-time.

New schemes to promote flexible training and working

The 'Improving Working Lives' initiative included new policies to allow doctors to have career breaks or periods outside full-time work. It was also seen as a retention initiative, resulting in improvements in the service to patients. The Flexible Career Scheme (FCS) provided central funding for hospital doctors and GPs who wanted to work less than half-time or for doctors planning to return to medicine. The scheme was available for doctors at all stages of their careers, including those who would have retired otherwise.

'Shifting the Balance of Power' is the name given by the government to a programme designed to move decision-making in the NHS to local levels, where services are delivered to patients. This programme has resulted in the increasing devolvement of central funding to strategic health authorities (SHAs), to primary care trusts (PCTs) and to deaneries. In the financial year 2005/2006 funding for the FCS became cash-limited and was devolved to SHAs and PCTs, which will significantly restrict access to the scheme in future years. Deaneries will need to prioritise eligibility to join the scheme, taking into account the needs of patients and the NHS as well as individual doctors.

Flexible training was first introduced in the 1970s in order to retain doctors who would otherwise have left the profession. New flexible training arrangements for hospital doctors were introduced in June 2005[19,20] to reflect the increasing demand for part-time training. Salaries are proportional to work actually done, with the aim of making flexible trainees mainstream rather than supernumerary by slot-sharing or working part-time in a full-time post. Trusts will need to look innovatively at their rotas in order to incorporate flexible training and the new arrangements require every trust to have 20% of its trainees working flexibly within five years, subject to demand.

Summary

The pressure from doctors to improve their work–life balance will continue to increase. White, male doctors no longer dominate the profession, and traditional ways of working will not be able to deliver the type of service required by the NHS for the benefit of patients. Further changes will be required to working patterns for doctors in training, including redesigning services to minimise night work.[21] Opportunities for flexible working after training has been completed are equally important but financial constraints must not be used as an excuse for stifling change to working patterns. In fact, new ways of working are even more imperative when funding is limited to ensure a high standard of healthcare delivery.

References

1   Griffiths E (2003) Just who are tomorrow's doctors? *BMJ Careers*. **326**: 4.

2   Department of Health (2001) *Improving Working Lives Standard*. Department of Health, London.

3   Department of Health (2003) *The European Working Time Directive, Guidance*. Department of Health, London.

4   Allen I (1988) *Doctors and their Careers*. Policy Studies Institute, London.

5   Allen I (1992) *Part-time Working in General Practice*. Policy Studies Institute, London.

6   Allen I (1994) *Doctors and their Careers: a new generation*. Policy Studies Institute, London.

7   Davidson JM, Lambert TW and Goldacre MJ (1998) Career pathways and destinations 18 years on among doctors who qualified in the United Kingdom in 1977: postal questionnaire survey. *BMJ*. **317**: 1425–1428.

8   Lambert TW and Goldacre MJ (1998) Career destinations seven years on among doctors who qualified in the United Kingdom in 1988: postal questionnaire survey. *BMJ*. **317**: 1429–1431.

9   NHS Executive (2000) *A Health Service of All the Talents: developing the NHS workforce*. Department of Health, London.

10 Parkhouse J (1991) *Doctors' Careers*. Routledge, London.

11 British Medical Association (2001) *BMA Cohort Study of 1995 Medical Graduates, Sixth Report*. BMA, London.

12 Secretary of State for Health (2000) *The NHS Plan – A Plan for Investment, A Plan for Reform*. Department of Health, London.

13 Department of Health (2002) *Improving Working Lives for Doctors*. Department of Health, London.

14   Lambert TW, Davidson JM, Evans J *et al*. (2003) Doctors' reasons for rejecting initial choice of specialties as long-term careers. *Medical Education*. **37**: 312–318.

15   Department of Health (2003) *The Response of the Four UK Health Ministers to the Consultation on Unfinished Business: proposals for reform of the House Officer grade*. Department of Health, London.

16   Sir Liam Donaldson, CMO (2002) *Unfinished Business: proposals for reform of the House Officer grade*. Department of Health, London.

17   Central Consultants and Specialist Committee (2003) *Job Planning: a summary for consultants new to the 2003 contract in England and Northern Ireland*. British Medical Association, London.

18   British Medical Association (2003) *New GMS Contract 2003: investing in general practice*. BMA Publications, London.

19   NHS Employers (2005) *Doctors in Flexible Training: equitable pay for flexible medical training*. NHS Employers, Leeds.

20   NHS Employers (2005) *Doctors in Flexible Training: principles underpinning the new arrangements for flexible training*. NHS Employers, Leeds.

21   www.modern.nhs.uk/hospitalatnight

CHAPTER 2

Flexible training in secondary care

Beverley Gainey

Introduction

'Less-than-full-time' training, as it is known in Scotland, or 'flexible training', as it is more commonly known in other regions, is one of a number of initiatives that recognises and supports the work–life balance for doctors in training. It is intended to provide a means to work less than full-time for those who need it, to enable those trainees to access effective training and to enable trusts to employ them in order that they can contribute to service delivery. Trainees who need to avail themselves of flexible training in order to achieve a satisfactory work–life balance represent a valuable resource in terms of investment to date and future service provision.

Flexible training enables doctors to reduce their working week by as much as half. The exact proportions favoured vary markedly between deaneries: six sessions can be a stipulated minimum or a stipulated maximum, where a session is equivalent to four hours. The majority of trainees work 60% of full-time.

Background

Without prejudice to the principle of full-time training as set out in Article 24(1) (c), and until such time as the Council takes decisions in accordance with paragraph 3, member states may permit part-time specialist training, under conditions approved by the competent national authorities, when training on a full-time basis would not be practicable for well-founded reasons. (EC Directive 93/16/EEC/Article 25)

In 1993, European legislation (Council Directive 93/16 EEC) pronounced that doctors in member states could train on a less-than-full-time basis when it was not practicable for well-founded reasons for them to do so on a full-time basis; however, 'well-founded reasons' was not actually defined. Flexible trainees have traditionally been supernumerary employees and deaneries have contributed to their salary costs in much the same way as they do for full-time trainees. As the budget for flexible training is one of a number competing for funding, it may be insufficient to meet all demands for flexible training in some regions at some times. To recognise and prioritise the different reasons behind requests to train flexibly, a 'Category I' and 'Category II' classification has been developed. 'Category I' trainees are those whose health or disabilities are such that it is not practicable for them to work and train on a full-time basis, or they have a carer's role, which places the same limitations upon their ability to work full-time, or, and much more commonly, they have child-care responsibilities that impinge upon their desire or ability to work full-time. It should be noted that recent parliamentary legislation (Employment Act 2002 part IV) imposed a legal obligation on employers to give reasonable consideration to a request for part-time working by any employee with a child under six. By default, all other applicants for flexible training are 'Category II'. In recent years deaneries have had to restrict flexible training to 'Category I' applicants because they have not had sufficient funding for both categories.

Implementation

Each deanery has a website that provides details of how the flexible training arrangements operate in their particular area. Doctors moving from one deanery to another need to be aware that they have to reapply to the new deanery, and that flexible training arrangements affecting them may vary. Most deaneries have an Associate Dean for flexible training, but other management arrangements also exist. Flexible training is available to all the medical training grades, but there are some practical differences between the grades, just as there are some practical differences between the deaneries in the operational arrangements for flexible training.

Flexible training should be an accurate reflection of full-time training, but on a pro rata basis. Flexible trainees should participate in all the medical activities carried out by the department where they work, including on-call duties in the evenings and weekends. They should be prepared and expect that they will be required to work at any time of the week and at any time of the year, in the same way as their full-time colleagues. This does not preclude trainees making local arrangements for particular fixed working patterns where these can be accommodated without prejudicing training and continuity of service delivery. However, if a trainee is unable to fulfil the basic requirement of availability on a regular basis, it may be that flexible training is inappropriate at this stage of their career. In other words, both employers and trainees must be flexible to a reasonable degree.

All flexible trainees must obtain a suitable training post or a placement on a suitable rotation in open competition. There are relatively few substantive part-time posts to apply for. Trainees wishing to work flexibly should apply for full-time posts but are not obliged to declare a need to work flexibly until after they have been successful at interview. In theory, and, it is hoped, in practice, advance knowledge that one or more candidates want to train flexibly will have no impact on the outcome of the recruitment process.

Placements

Once a doctor has obtained a suitable post in open competition, he or she may be accommodated in one of three different types of placement. The flexible trainee may work reduced sessions in a full-time post; alternatively, the flexible trainee may share that full-time post with another flexible trainee; lastly, though not available in all deaneries at present, there may be the opportunity to have a supernumerary placement. Working on their own in, or sharing, a substantive full-time post will generally provide a better educational experience than being supernumerary. Being more than another additional pair of hands, the training experience derived from occupying a substantive post is more easily a proportional reflection of the full-time trainee, as the trainee is participating in mainstream training.

Sharing a post with another trainee in the flexible training sense, known as 'slot-sharing' in some deaneries, does not mean that the salary and responsibilities are divided equally between the two individuals. Rather, both trainees can work up to the maximum number of sessions allowed in their particular deanery, and they are paid as individuals. The two flexible trainees may work very closely together, with involved handovers to ensure continuity of patient care, or, at the other extreme, they may be based on different sites with little service need to interact very much at all. The way the slot-share works in practice will depend on the nature and content of the full-time post. Funding arrangements for slot-share arrangements also vary between deaneries.

Early planning will help to get the optimum return from a flexible training placement. For example, in a slot-share arrangement that is anticipated to be of a year's duration, it may be advantageous from a training perspective for slot-sharers to work one half of the week for the first six months, and then to swap over for the second six months. Flexible trainees should find out the opportunities for structured training at the trust where they will be working and incorporate these into their working week if possible. The flexible trainee's working week should resemble that of a full-time trainee as closely as possible, on a proportional basis.

Subject to being eligible, training capacity and funding being available and a satisfactory service commitment, trainees can move in and out of flexible training to suit their changing needs. They can do so for short or long periods, intersperse full-time training with a number of periods of flexible training and increase or decrease their hours. In reality it may take quite some time to organise the required placement changes, due to the timing of rotations, other trainees' needs and service requirements, but the spirit of the flexible training concept is that all parties are as flexible as they can be.

At the completion of training, the quantity and quality of an individual's training should not differ between trainees who have trained full-time, flexibly or in combinations of the two, other than periods of flexible training will lengthen the overall training period. Flexible trainees will therefore need to rotate in the same way as their full-time colleagues, and must undertake pro rata out-of-hours and on-call duties. Unless the circumstances that justify flexible training make this impossible, flexible trainees should not train for more than six months without out-of-hours or on-call commitments when it would be normal in their stage of training and speciality to do so.

The notion that flexible trainees can select or even dictate where they wish to train has given rise to the belief that flexible training offers the opportunity to 'cherry-pick' placements. This should not be the case, and the reasonable consideration of flexible trainees' needs should not be at the expense of full-time trainees. For example, a flexible trainee could not reasonably expect to avoid having to rotate to the trusts involving the longest travelling time simply because they were training flexibly if a full-time trainee would be expected to do so regardless of their child or carer commitments. If something is difficult to cope with for a few days a week, having to do so full-time will be more difficult, and it is worth remembering that full-time trainees have families and health issues, too.

It should be noted that where funding is available to support supernumerary placements, there is no intended implication that this enables flexible trainees to have their choice of any placement on a scheme; a more valid interpretation is that supernumerary funding is a stop-gap arrangement where there has been a failure to identify an opportunity to occupy, individually or paired, a substantive post.[1]

Application

The application process starts with an approach to the deanery responsible for the trusts in the area the doctor wishes to work in. Depending on the deanery approached, the doctor will either have an interview with the Associate Dean for flexible training (Postgraduate Dean in Scotland), or be sent an eligibility form to complete. If the doctor is not already working within the grade and specialty, he or she will need to secure a post in open competition. If the deanery has given the doctor approval to train flexibly then the doctor can declare this before, at or after interview.If deanery approval has not been sought and granted before-hand, the applicant to the post will not be able to start flexible training until this approval has been properly obtained. In the meantime the applicant can accept the whole-time post, not work, or perhaps continue in their present post where this has not been filled already.

If the deanery has declined to approve a trainee for flexible training for some reason, and the junior doctor wishes to appeal against that decision, there is an appeals process. This may vary from deanery to deanery, but will be broadly in line with the process outlined in the document issued by the NHS Employers entitled 'Principles underpinning the new arrangements for flexible training';[2] this can be viewed on their website (www.nhsemployers.org).

Educational approval

All flexible training placements must have educational approval, and this should be in place before the flexible trainee starts the placement. Foundation Year 1 and Foundation Year 2 (F1 and F2) flexible trainees can contact their Foundation School Director for advice on their proposed flexible training programme. The Postgraduate Medical Education and Training Board (PMETB) approves the foundation programmes on the recommendation of the Postgraduate Dean and Foundation School. If already working in a foundation programme then preliminary advice should be obtained from the local training programme director or clinical tutor in the individual trust. For specialty training placements, doctors can approach the chair of the Specialist or Higher Training Committee, the specialty programme director or the flexible training specialty advisers, who will know the particular Royal College requirements for their specialty.

Academic medicine

Requests for flexible training for medical academics (lecturer or clinical lecturer positions) are handled in the same way as for other medical trainees, and they need to meet the same criteria. Doctors in full-time academic training posts who wish to train flexibly for well-founded reasons may be able to continue in their current post on a reduced number of sessions if practicable given the service component of that individual post. Alternatively, they relinquish their substantive post and become supernumerary, releasing the full-time training opportunity. The academic unit providing the training would need to agree the management of the overall training opportunities with the relevant Postgraduate Dean and Speciality Training Committee.

Doctors who are already training flexibly and are minded to take an academic placement may, with the support of senior academic staff in their specialty, be considered for regrading as part-time clinical lecturers. They would continue to hold their national training number (NTN) and as an honorary specialist trainee they would continue in a training programme towards their certificate of completion of training (CCT), with funding from the flexible training budget as appropriate.

Undertaking research is not generally considered sufficient reason to train on a flexible basis, as opportunities for research can ordinarily be accommodated within the full-time training programme.

Period of grace

The period of grace, whereby a trainee can continue in the specialty training grade for up to six months post-CCT, is also available to flexible trainees, but it should be noted that the period allowed is six calendar months and not six months' equivalent on a pro rata basis.

Summary

The demand for flexible training rises each year and accounted for 6% of trainees in 2005. Flexible training is included in the Trust Educational Contract as one of the Department of Health's *Improving Working Lives Standard*[3] and requires trusts to increase this figure to 20% by 2010, subject to demand. Flexible training will need to become increasingly mainstream and this will only happen with a change in attitude by employing trusts.

Flexible training is not an easy option, and it takes time, patience, negotiating skills and resilience to organise. There should be plenty of help and advice available but it remains the primary responsibility of trainees to organise their flexible training.

References

1 NHS Employers (2005) *Doctors in Flexible Training: equitable pay for flexible medical training.* NHS Employers, Leeds.

2 NHS Employers (2005) *Doctors in Flexible Training: principles underpinning the new arrangements for flexible training.* NHS Employers, Leeds.

3 Department of Health (2001) *Improving Working Lives Standard.* Department of Health, London.

CHAPTER 3

Flexible training for general practice

Anne Hastie

Introduction

Modernising Medical Careers[1] (MMC) introduced a new training programme (a foundation programme) starting in August 2005 for the first two years of a doctor's postgraduate training. A run-through programme of specialty training starting in August 2007, which for general practice takes three years, follows this. In addition there may be the opportunity to undertake two years of in-service higher professional education (HPE) on completion of specialty general practice training. MMC has created the opportunity to improve general practice training, making it more flexible and competency-based.

General practice is an ideal career for doctors who want to work part-time or have flexible working arrangements. The training is not as long as other specialties and the lifetime earnings of general practitioners (GPs) are relatively higher than those of many hospital colleagues. General practice is increasingly becoming a first choice of career for new doctors and the introduction of placements in general practice during foundation programmes is expected to attract more doctors into general practice. Doctors can choose to enter a three-year run-through specialty training programme for general practice on completion of their foundation programme or, alternatively, those who have not decided on a their final career choice may be able to join a generic specialty training programme and then transfer to complete a final two years in a general practice training programme. However, this is subject to further review by the Royal College of General Practitioners (RCGP) and the Postgraduate Medical Education and Training Board (PMETB).

Female doctors who initially plan a hospital career sometimes decide to change to general practice once they have children because it has family-friendly ways of working. If they have several years of experience in a hospital specialty the time will not be wasted as their skills can be transferred to general practice, where they can become a practitioner with special interest (PwSI). Skills in specialties such as dermatology, cardiology, gynaecology and surgery are particularly attractive to practices and can generate additional practice income.

This chapter will describe the various aspects of the three-year specialty training for general practice, including flexible training. However, changes are likely to occur to the various processes involved in general practice training and doctors are advised to keep up to date by visiting appropriate websites for more information:

- Royal College of General Practitioners (www.rcgp.org.uk)
- Postgraduate Medical Education Training Board (www.pmetb.org.uk)
- *Modernising Medical Careers* (www.mmc.nhs.uk)
- Postgraduate deaneries (e.g. www.londondeanery.ac.uk).

Regulatory framework

On 30 September 2005 the PMETB assumed the functions of the Joint Committee on Postgraduate Training for General Practice (JCPTGP). The RCGP became responsible for processing applications for certificates on behalf of the PMETB. The RCGP charges a fee for processing applications and the PMETB charges a fee for certification. The PMETB certificate is the legal licence to work as a GP in the UK. Doctors must register with the RCGP in order to obtain an assessment of their eligibility for a certificate and they will receive free associate membership from the time of their registration.

Doctors must also join the Performer List of their primary care organisation (PCO) before being eligible to work in general practice, and this includes GP registrars. The PCO will check:

- the PMETB (or JCPTGP) certificate (except for GP registrars)
- General Medical Council (GMC) registration
- Criminal Records Bureau (CRB) check
- clinical references
- medical indemnity insurance.

Certificate of Completion of Training

This used to be called a 'Certificate of Prescribed Experience' and was issued by the JCPTGP. However, the framework for general practice training is now defined by the PMETB under Article 10 of the *Order*.[2] In order to complete specialist training for general practice trainees must do at least three years' full-time training or equivalent part-time within a seven-year period preceding their application for a 'Certificate of Completion of Training' (CCT).[3]

The training programme must include:

- 12 months in an approved training practice with an approved GP trainer
- 12 months in other specialties approved for GP training
- 12 months in combinations of the above.

It is hoped that as much of the training as possible, and 18 months at least, will be based in primary care but this is subject to available funding. The PMETB needs to be satisfied that the overall training programme is well balanced.

List A specialties

A maximum of 12 months' full-time or equivalent part-time in any of the following specialties can count towards GP training. This list may be reviewed and altered by the PMETB in the future.

- Accident and Emergency (A&E) medicine
- paediatrics or community paediatrics
- general medicine, geriatrics, dermatology, genitourinary medicine or rehabilitation medicine
- gynaecology or obstetrics and gynaecology (O&G)
- psychiatry or old age psychiatry
- palliative medicine.

The three-year training programme must include:

- at least six months in each of two List A specialties, or
- at least four months in three List A specialties, or
- at least three months in four List A specialties.

List B specialties

Providing the overall programme is well balanced the PMETB may also accept training of up to six months' full-time or equivalent part-time in List B specialties towards a CCT. Individual trainees should obtain an assessment of their proposed training programme from the RCGP if they want to include a List B specialty, such as:

- cardiology, oncology, gastroenterology, endocrinology, rheumatology, neurology or infectious diseases
- child and adolescent psychiatry or psychiatry of learning disabilities
- ophthalmology, ears, nose and throat (ENT), general or paediatric surgery, urology, trauma and orthopaedics
- intensive care medicine
- public health medicine.

Statement of eligibility for registration (Article 11)

This used to be covered by the JCPTGP as a 'Certificate of Equivalent Experience'. Doctors whose training does not comply with Article 10 can have their experience assessed under Article 11. A doctor's experience might include:

- trust posts, such as working as a clinical fellow
- training abroad
- work as an overseas GP
- training done more than seven years ago.

If training is more than seven years ago applicants must show they have been working in clinical medicine without significant breaks. Applicants should register with the RCGP Certification Unit, which will require detailed information about the experience being submitted, and approval is not guaranteed. Fees will be charged by the RCGP and the PMETB for making an assessment of any experience being submitted under Article 11.

Curriculum for general practice training

The RCGP has produced a new curriculum for GP training and full details are available on the website (www.rcgp.org.uk). The curriculum is competency-based with an emphasis on learning in the workplace, supervision and assessment. The curriculum covers the core GP skills,[4] which are:

- primary care management
- person-centred care
- specific GP problem-solving skills
- a comprehensive approach
- community orientation
- a holistic approach.

Application process

Doctors are appointed to GP training programmes through a national recruitment process. Advertisements appear in the *British Medical Journal* (BMJ) and the following training opportunities are available in most deaneries:

- three-year vocational training schemes (VTS)
- shortened vocational training schemes (usually two years or 18 months) for doctors who have already done some training that can count towards their CCT

- GP registrar posts for doctors who have constructed their own GP training or are required by the PMETB to do a GP registrar post under Article 11.

Deaneries use various methods to help with their selection process, which may include:

- competency questions
- multiple choice questions (MCQs)
- group exercises
- written exercises
- patient simulation
- central interviews.

It is probable that all deaneries will eventually use the same selection process, but there are organisational difficulties for deaneries that have a large number of applicants and posts.

Doctors who wish to train flexibly should check their eligibility with the relevant deanery and then apply through the national recruitment process in the same way as those wishing to train full-time. All members of interview panels are trained in equal opportunities and will not be told that the applicant plans to train flexibly. If an applicant is successful at interview and offered a VTS or GP registrar post they should then declare their wish to train flexibly. Deaneries will give guidance on organising flexible training but a placement is subject to an employer being willing to employ the doctor on a flexible basis and individual doctors are responsible for organising their flexible training placement.

Self-constructing general practice training

Some doctors choose to construct their own training programme for general practice training but this is becoming increasingly difficult as a lot of stand-alone posts have been allocated to foundation programmes or run-through specialty training. If a doctor has approval for flexible training funding they must still obtain a post in open competition before asking to train flexibly. They cannot have a post created for them just because they have the required funding agreement.

Open competition means that a vacant post is appropriately advertised in media such as the *BMJ*, websites and e-mail. The principle is to bring the vacancy to the attention of as many potential applicants as possible who may consider that they meet the criteria for the job and satisfy the published person specification. After the closing date applicants are considered by a panel for short-listing in accordance with an objective, transparent and fair system drawn from the person specification, and considered specifically against these criteria alone. Using these criteria, the highest-ranked applicants using these criteria will be short-listed; the interview process should also be such that the ranking and selection of applicants can be justified against the objective criteria set out in the person specification.

Flexible training in hospital posts

The EEC directive for the training of GPs requires trainees to work at least one week full-time during the hospital component of their training. A good week to choose is the first week of a post, when the hospital and departmental induction is taking place. The rest of the training must be at least 50% of full-time, although training done before 31 October 2002 must have been at least 60% of full-time. Many deaneries will only fund flexible training up to 80% of full-time and expect those who want to work more than 80% to work full-time. New flexible training arrangements ensures that the pay for a hospital flexible trainee is proportional to the full-time pay.[5] The employing trust and not the deanery funds any out-of-hours payments.

The timetable of the flexible trainee should be based on the full-time timetable of trainees in the same grade and the same department.[6] All parts of the post should be done at the same agreed percentage of:

- daytime work
- educational activities
- on-call
- out-of-hours.

A maximum of six months' training can be completed without out-of-hours in special circumstances. Doctors who are breastfeeding are exempt from out-of-hours but they need to check this will not affect the educational approval of their post.

Trainees who want to work flexibly usually have to organise their own hospital training posts, with help from the deanery and the local VTS course organisers. Under the new flexible training arrangements[6] trusts will be expected to employ 5% of their doctors flexibly in 2005/2006 rising to 20% in 2010/2011, subject to demand and trusts will be performance managed on these percentages. Flexible trainees can be employed by trusts in the following ways.

Slot-shares

The deanery already funds 50% of full-time posts approved for GP training. Each slot-sharer can work more than five sessions and the deanery can choose to fund the additional costs over the normal full-time post. For example, if two slot-sharers work 80% each (160% in total) the deanery can choose to fund the additional 60%.

Supernumerary posts

For supernumerary posts the deanery funds the daytime sessions worked, for example five sessions for 50% flexible trainees, six sessions for 60%, etc., and the trust funds the additional costs associated with any additional hours of actual work and the out-of-hours supplement. Some deaneries will only fund up to six sessions.

Reduced sessions in a full-time post

Full-time posts are already 50% funded by the deanery even if no one is in post. If a department has a vacant full-time post, this should be used instead of a supernumerary placement.

If flexible trainees are working as a job-share or part-time in a full-time post educational approval should already be in place. However, if a supernumerary post is being created using flexible training funding educational approval must be obtained on an ad personam basis before starting in post. This will require the submission of details of the post to the Director of Postgraduate General Practice Education (DPGPE), including:

- a completed PMETB Form B (GP) 'Application for the approval of a training post'
- personal development plan (PDP) for the post
- clinical timetable
- educational timetable, including attendance at the VTS half-day
- name of the educational supervisor
- percentage of full-time.

The deanery GP Education and Training Committee (or equivalent) then ratifies educational approval. The PMETB Form B (GP), supporting evidence and a covering letter from the DPGPE is then sent to the PMETB for final approval.

There are imaginative ways that trusts could employ flexible trainees for general practice in consultation with their deanery:

- Two doctors slot-share a full-time post and a third flexible trainee is supernumerary. If one of the slot-sharers leaves the supernumerary trainee moves into the slot-share until a replacement is found.
- A flexible trainee works reduced sessions in a full-time post. Under the new flexible pay agreement sufficient money should be left over for the trust to make other arrangements to cover service provision.

Table 3.1: Calculations for reduced sessions in a full-time post

Percentage worked	Part-time training for a 12-month full-time post	Part-time training for a 6-month full-time post
50%	24 months	12 months
60%	20 months	10 months
66.66%	18 months	9 months
75%	16 months	8 months
80%	15 months	7.5 months
85%	14.1 months (56 weeks and 3 days)	7.05 months (28 weeks and 1.5 days)
90%	13.3 months (53 weeks and 2 days)	6.6 months (26 weeks and 4 days)
95%	12.6 months (50 weeks and 4 days)	6.3 months (25 weeks and 2 days)
100%	12 months	6 months

- Trusts can advertise for two slot-sharers to fill a full-time post.
- If there is a slot-share and one person leaves the remaining slot-sharer can become supernumerary so the trust can fill the post with a full-time trainee or employ a locum while advertising for a replacement slot-sharer.
- By employing slot-sharers who work more than 100% (it could be two sharers doing 80% = 160%) the trust may be able to lower the banding for the other trainees in the department, making cost-savings. This solution does require advanced planning, as it would affect full-time contracts.

Part-time training as a GP registrar

The budget for funding GP registrar posts is the same for full- and part-time posts, unlike hospital training where there is a separate budget for flexible training. A placement is subject to a GP trainer being willing to employ a part-time GP registrar but this is rarely a problem as practices like having a doctor who will be with them for more than one year. Training as a GP registrar can be on a 'non-continuous' basis subject to approval by the DPGPE.

GP registrars must work at least 50% of full-time, and work at least one week full-time during their general practice placement. The timetable should be based on what a full-time GP registrar works in the same practice. The regulations require a part-time GP registrar to work the same percentage of clinical sessions, educational sessions, on-call and out-of-hours. The GP registrar cannot reduce the number of clinical sessions but continue with a 100% of educational activities. At the end of their part-time training period they should have completed the same amount of training as a full-time GP registrar.

One session equates to four hours and a full-time working week comprises 10 sessions, which equates to 40 hours per week plus out-of-hours (pro rata for part-time). A typical full-time GP registrar timetable might include:

- seven clinical sessions
- one session to attend the VTS educational half-day
- one flexible, planned educational session
- one session for a tutorial.

The timetable will vary according to local arrangements, for example a VTS educational full-day, but it is important that GP registrars get sufficient clinical experience. Although a session should be four hours it is recognised that some sessions may be longer while others shorter, but the overall full-time working week should be 40 hours plus out-of-hours. GP registrars and trainers should therefore look at the total workload/hours rather than the hours of an individual session.

VTS course organisers like GP registrars to attend every week to avoid disruption. A part-time GP registrar could choose to attend every week for a year and then do other activities for the remainder of their training. If they want to continue going to the VTS it should be at the expense of other educational activities such as the flexible session. For example, a GP registrar working 50% might choose to go to the VTS during term time and have their flexible session during the academic holidays. Some degree of flexibility around educational activities is acceptable providing it is at the appropriate percentage and supports the GP registrar's learning needs.

Out-of-hours experience for GP registrars

The new GP contract makes a clear distinction between normal general practice and out-of-hours care. The wide range of out-of-hours provisions now available means that GP registrars need to gain sufficient experience of the different settings where out-of-hours takes place.[7] There are a number of organisations involved in the delivery of out-of-hours care, including NHS Direct, GP co-ops, commercial deputising services, minor injury centres, primary care walk-in centres and accident and emergency departments. Every model of service has a place in general practice training and a flexible approach is required to meet the varying educational needs of individual GP registrars.

A number of core skills and competencies can be identified that are necessary for the performance of out-of-hours care, and GP registrars should be equipped with these competencies on completing training regardless of their intentions relating to future provision of out-of-hours care. Experience during the GP registrar's training period should be directed towards the attainment of these competencies. Out-of-hours care should be specifically addressed within the initial assessment of a GP registrar's learning needs and be revisited through formative assessment with the aim of developing confidence and competence in this area.

Sessions in out-of-hours

Out-of-hours is normally considered to mean medical care delivered at weekends, bank holidays and between 6.30 pm and 8 am on weekdays. When arranging out-of-hours experience, GP registrars and their trainers should note the following guidance.

- The duration and frequency of sessions worked by a GP registrar will vary depending on their nature, but normally a 4–6 hour session every four weeks would be appropriate.
- A full-time GP registrar is expected to undertake a minimum of 12 such sessions during one year and part-time is pro rata.
- A GP registrar who works an overnight session should have the following day off.
- Out-of-hours work should not be undertaken the night before any organised educational activity.
- The GP registrar should maintain a log of all out-of-hours sessions.
- Appropriate educational supervision must be available for all out-of-hours sessions and GP registrars must be aware at all times of how to access this provision.
- GP registrars do not receive additional payment for out-of-hours work as their salary already includes a substantial out-of-hours pay component.
- In undertaking out-of-hours sessions, GP registrars should ensure that adequate indemnity arrangements are in place to cover their own individual circumstances.

Innovative training posts

Deaneries have been developing innovative training posts (ITPs) using GP registrar funding. Trainees are employed by a training practice and have a GP trainer as their educational supervisor. A typical post will be based on a PDP with 40% of the time spent in general practice and 60% in attachments to secondary care or community specialties. An evaluation of innovative training posts was very positive[8] and compared favourably to the traditional senior house officer (SHO) post, because it was planned for a future career in general practice. The sessions in secondary or community care may involve ward work, outpatients and community clinics. Trainees may need to gain experience in the acute care of the specialty, which should include on-call. Out-of-hours work may involve primary care sessions or a contribution to the acute trust's out-of-hours provision.

Limited funding for GP registrar placements makes it unlikely that many doctors will be able to do more than one innovative training post.

Assessments

Doctors undertaking general practice training have to pass summative assessment (SA), which includes an MCQ, assessment of consulting skills, a written piece of work and a structured trainer's report in order to obtain their JCPTGP certificate. In addition, many GP registrars choose to do the examinations for membership of the Royal College of General Practitioners (MRCGP). The PMETB is committed to reducing the burden of assessment so SA and the MRCGP examinations will possibly be replaced by one assessment package, based on three components:

- workplace-based assessment throughout the three years
- a machine-marked test of applied knowledge
- clinical skills assessment.

Successful completion of the assessments will result in the qualification nMRCGP.

Transitional arrangements will be in place until August 2007, but doctors who complete general practice training after August 2007 will have to do the new MRCGP assessment. Satisfactory completion of the three components by the end of a three-year general practice training programme will make the candidate eligible for their CCT and nMRCGP. If a doctor fails any of the components he or she can apply for an extension to their GP registrar placement, which will normally be granted for an additional six months.

Absence during training for general practice

The regulations allow up to one week of leave during any six-month GP registrar period of training for sickness, maternity, adoption and paternity leave but absence in excess of this must be made up by extending the GP registrar contract. During a two-year hospital programme absences up to one month (pro rata for shorter periods of training) will not normally be expected to be made up. If the absence is for a longer time it must be made up but not necessarily in the specialty or post where the absence occurred.[9] DPGPEs can use their discretion if absences exceed the guidelines by a small amount. In many cases it is possible to extend the GP registrar contract to cover relatively short absences during hospital training. Trainees need to check with the RCGP/PMETB that their plans to make up lost time comply with the regulations.

Summary

It has become increasingly popular to do general practice training on a part-time basis but it does require advance planning by the individual doctor, particularly during the hospital component of their training. Regulations, guidance and opportunities can change so it is important that doctors obtain up-to-date information on a regular basis and seek help if problems arise. General practice is a rewarding career for those who want to work part-time and/or flexibly, and it is worth the effort to complete their training and gain a CCT and MRCGP.

References

1 Department of Health (2003) *Modernising Medical Careers. The Response of the Four UK Health Ministers to the Consultation of Unfinished Business: proposals for reform of the House Officer grade.* Department of Health, London.

2 Postgraduate Medical Education and Training Board (2003) *The General and Specialist Medical Practice (Education, Training and Qualifications) Order.* The Stationery Office, London.

3 Royal College of General Practitioners (2005) *PMETB Certificate of Completion of Training.* RCGP, London.

4 Deighan M and Field S (2005) *Specialist Training for General Practice Newsletter: a guide to the new GP curriculum.* RCGP, London.

5 NHS Employers (2005) *Doctors in Flexible Training: equitable pay for flexible medical training.* NHS Employers, Leeds.

6 NHS Employers (2005) *Doctors in Flexible Training: principles underpinning the new arrangements for flexible training.* NHS Employers, Leeds.

7 COGPED (2004) *Out of Hours (OOH) Training for GP Registrars: position paper (including DH guidance).* COGPED, London.

8 Field N, Mather N and Lane P (2002) Innovative training posts in general practice: an evaluation of the North Trent experience. *Education for Primary Care.* **13**: 362–370.

9 Joint Committee on Postgraduate Training for General Practice (2004) *A Guide to Certification.* JCPTGP, London.

CHAPTER 4

Flexible working and training for dentists

Elizabeth Jones and Anne Hastie

Introduction

An increasing proportion of the dental workforce is female and it is predicted that by 2020 over 50% of practising dentists will be women.[1] In October 2000 just over 50% of UK dental schools entrants were female. Dentists of both sexes are becoming increasingly interested in part-time and/or flexible working patterns as they seek a better work–life balance. Dentistry is a perfect career for those who want to train and work part-time. Although on-call commitments are necessary in many branches of medicine, the on-call commitments in dentistry are minimal, which suits those for whom part-time training and working is important. Employers are beginning to understand that recruitment and retention of female dentists depends on flexible working opportunities.

In 2000 the Department of Health commissioned a review of employment opportunities for women dentists in the National Health Service (NHS).[2] The review was initiated because:

- fifty per cent of women in dentistry worked no more than two days per week in the NHS
- most women chose to work as associates in general dental services or as salaried dentists in community dental services
- the perception was that women found it difficult to return to dentistry after taking a career break.

Dame Margaret Seward was the author of this excellent report,[2] which was based on an extensive postal questionnaire, focus groups and responses from individuals and professional organisations. It was published in 2001 and made many suggestions for improving the working lives of dentists, including the appointment of retaining and returning advisers. The report found that although dentists perceived a problem in getting part-time work this was not the reality, and 92% of those who wanted part-time work were successful in finding suitable employment.

Other drivers for change included the Department of Health 'Improving Working Lives' campaign[3] and employment legislation on the rights to request flexible working.[4] The NHS is undergoing rapid change and dentists are having to adapt to new contracts. Up to date information is available on several websites, including the following.

- British Dental Association (www.bda-dentistry.org.uk)
- General Dental Council (www.gdc-uk.org)
- Department of Health (www.dh.gov.uk).

The most common reasons for dentists choosing to work part-time in 2000 (may be more than one reason for each dentist) were:[2]

- caring for children (65%)
- personal choice (57%)
- ill-health (4%)
- working outside dentistry (4%)
- caring for a relative (3%).

This chapter discusses the various options for flexible training and working in the NHS, although it is recognised that many dentists choose to work in private practice. Only 5% of female dentists hold a university appointment – because of the lack of flexibility and career pathways which are based on traditional working patterns.[2] This is further explored in Chapter 12.

Postgraduate flexible training for dentists

There are two aspects of flexible training to be considered:

- vocational training for general dental practitioners
- training leading to entry on to a specialist list.

Vocational training

To obtain a primary care trust (PCT) number in order to work in NHS general dental practice UK graduates are required to undertake a year in vocational training. The aims of vocational training for general dental service are to meet the needs of unsupervised general dental practice by developing the clinical skills learnt as an undergraduate and teaching administrative and practice management skills to promote high ethical standards and quality care for patients. By the end of the vocational training period, the vocational dental practitioner should be eligible to practise unsupervised as a general dental practitioner within the general dental service.

Prospective vocational dental practitioners are responsible for obtaining two professional references, which can be from tutors at dental school and should comment on their clinical competency. The dentist must be registered with the General Dental Council (GDC) and be a member of a defence organisation before signing a vocational training contract, and, from 1 April 2006 must be on the PCT's Performers List. They cannot sign a contract until after they have passed their final dental examinations.

A requirement of the vocational training year is that trainees complete a specified number of hours in the practice and attend 30 study days. Each trainee belongs to a 'scheme' of approximately 12 vocational dental practitioners who meet their scheme vocational training adviser once a week for a study day. The programme for the study day follows a common curriculum but the content can vary from scheme to scheme.

Trainees can opt to train part-time for up to two years, usually at 50%. All the study days are attended within one year and the number of hours worked in the practice can be organised by negotiation between trainer and trainee. The total number of hours worked must be equivalent to that worked by a full-time vocational trainee. If training has been satisfactory at the end of the period of part-time training the vocational dental practitioner is given a certificate of satisfactory completion of vocational training.

Vocational training trainers

Carefully selected trainers, in inspected and approved practices, are chosen so that the vocational training year is as beneficial as possible. Postgraduate dental deaneries are always looking for new trainers and this role can be undertaken on a part-time basis. New trainers attend courses to prepare them for their supervisory and guiding roles, and experienced trainers should attend update courses on a regular basis. Trainers receive:

- a training grant
- reimbursement of the trainee's salary and employer's costs
- all fees earned by the vocational dental practitioner accrue to the practice.

Dental Vocational Training Authority

Before April 2006 dentists could apply to the Dental Vocational Training Authority (DVTA) for a vocational training number based on their experience and training if it was considered equivalent to dental vocational training. Application for a vocational training number through equivalent experience requires a considerable amount of detailed evidence. From April 2006 the Department of Health is introducing local commissioning of primary care dental services[5] and the functions of the DVTA will be reassigned, including the following:

- Delegating responsibility for determining equivalence of vocational training to PCTs but acting on the advice of the postgraduate dental deans.
- Transferring responsibility for award of a vocational training number to the new Business Services Authority.
- The DVTA set minimum guidelines on the criteria for trainer approval (http://cvtoffice.org.uk/vtinfo_dd1.htm), but from 1 April 2006 this responsibility is devolved to PCTs and postgraduate dental deans.

Training leading to entry on to a specialist list

At the time of writing there are specialist training programmes in all branches of dentistry. These include:

- orthodontics
- restorative dentistry
- monospecialties of periodontics, prosthodontics and endodontics
- paediatric dentistry
- dental public health
- additional dental specialties of oral pathology, oral medicine, oral microbiology and oral and maxillofacial radiology
- surgical dentistry
- academic oral surgery.

The specialist list review from the GDC (which is the sole competent authority for dentistry) went to consultation in December 2005 and it is likely that there will also be specialist lists opened in special needs dentistry and oral surgery. Oral and maxillofacial surgery is a postgraduate medical specialty rather than dental and is one of the nine recognised surgical specialties.

All trainees on specialist registrar (SpR) programmes fall under the terms and conditions of SpR training, which is the same as the medical specialties. The monospecialties are self-funded but are nevertheless governed by the terms and conditions of SpR training. As in the case of medical specialties any dental SpR can apply to train flexibly, and flexible training is covered in detail in Chapter 2. It can include slot-sharing, which means there is more than one trainee in a substantive post. Alternatively, there are some substantive posts which are advertised at SpR level as 'part-time'. This is usually because either the consultant in charge of training is part-time and cannot therefore supervise a trainee on a full-time basis, or because there is insufficient funding from the trust for a full-time appointment. In all types of flexible training, the timetable needs to be agreed by the specialist advisory committee (SAC) and the length of training decided upon. Appraisals and assessments will take place in the same way as for full-time trainees.

From a practical perspective flexible trainees are often in the minority, and because the numbers of trainees in some dental specialties are small, they may be a lone voice. It is therefore important that flexible trainees make regular contact with their educational supervisor to ensure that important lectures, seminars or didactic teaching, which may be programmed on days when part-time trainees are not scheduled to work, can be made up or attended with sessions taken in lieu. This must be the responsibility of flexible trainees working with their educational supervisor who, in turn, needs to work closely with the training programme director. Any issues pertaining to individual training requirements should be discussed at regular appraisals.

The length of SpR training varies between specialties and more information on the different curricula is available on www.rcseng.ac.uk/fds/training/documents.html.

Flexible working in dentistry

The main areas where dentists work in the NHS are:

- primary care
- community
- hospital.

Primary care dentistry

From April 2006 PCTs take over responsibility for commissioning primary care dental services within a national framework.[5] One of the aims of this reform is to improve the quality of dentists' working lives and this should include flexible working patterns.

All practising dentists will need to be on the PCT new dental Performers List from April 2006. Dentists who were previously associates will become performers and can safeguard their self-employed status by being paid on the basis of the work they actually do. Dentists should submit an invoice to their employing provider at the end of each month for units of dental activity (UDAs) they have completed, and they will receive varying payments each month according to their activity levels. In personal dental service practices some performers, who were previously associates, are paid fixed amounts each month for the service they provide and so they should be salaried employees.

Providers of dental services can be self-employed dentists who own the practice, or other providers who agree a contract with the PCT. There will be two main types of contracts for general dental practice:

- General dental services (GDS). Dentists will be offered a guaranteed NHS contract in return for an agreed level of NHS commitment spread over the year.

- Personal dental services (PDS) will allow dentists to provide more creative posts and the providers hold a practice-based contract as a group with the PCT. PDS practices are paid on the basis of their practice-based contract from an agreed budget providing they meet targets set by the PCT.

PDS has increased the availability of salaried posts, with a flexible policy towards working hours in some practices. If a performer leaves a PDS practice the contract and funding remains with the practice. However, a performer (including a previous associate) in a GDS practice is entitled to an individual provider contract from 1 April 2006, which could cause loss of income to the practice if they were to leave.

Out-of-hours

The 1990 contract for dentists required them to provide 24-hour emergency cover in NHS general dental practice. This was a deterrent for many female dentists because of safety fears or difficulty in arranging childcare. The new commissioning of dental services, due to be introduced in April 2006, gives responsibility for providing out-of-hours care to PCTs.[5] Dentists can agree to continue to provide out-of-hours care for the PCT under the new arrangements, but this is not compulsory.

Community dentistry

Community dental services provides dental care for patients with special needs, including young children, older people and patients with disabilities. It is a popular option for dentists wanting to work part-time as posts are salaried and there is a defined career structure, with opportunities for management and research.

Hospital dentistry

Hospital dentistry is less popular with doctors who want to work flexibly, and only a small proportion of women dentists reach senior positions in the hospital service.[2] Hospital dentists have the same employment structure and conditions of service as doctors (*see* Chapter 5). A new consultant contract was introduced in England in 2003 and this applies to all new consultants and those opting to change over from the old contract. The new contract is based on a programmed activity of four hours' duration (three hours if it is worked 'out of hours'). A full-time contract is for 10 programmed activities, although additional programmed activities are allowed for extra work. Therefore, a consultant, with the agreement of the trust, can work less than 10 programmed activities per week and be paid accordingly. It is possible, with the agreement of the trust/employer, to have a contract that varies throughout the year. This is particularly helpful for consultants who have other commitments that are variable, such as childcare, children's holiday cover or research. This new contract has greatly enhanced the ability to work part-time or flexibly, and often suits not only the consultant but also the trust.

Non-consultant career-grade dentists are responsible to a named dental consultant. The post is usually for a set commitment, based on service requirements, and this may be less than full-time and involve some flexibility, although this needs to be discussed with the employing trust. Usually these posts are filled by dentists who are committed to a career in hospital dentistry but who do not want to take on the responsibilities of a consultant, or those dentists who did not complete their specialist training.

Continuing professional development

Continuing professional development (CPD) is a mandatory requirement of the GDC for retention on the Dentists Register,[6] and the amount of CPD that has to be undertaken is the same whether a dentist works full- or part-time. The key features are:

- 250 hours of CPD over five years
- dentists maintain their own CPD record
- dentists submit an annual statement of the number of CPD hours they have completed each year
- the GDC monitors compliance by random sampling
- dentists who come off the register will have to complete all outstanding CPD before they can re-register.

Department of Health courses (previously known as Section 63)

The Department of Health allocates grants and pays fees to the providers of 'instruction conducive to the securing of the efficient provision of General Dental Services'. In England, responsibility for providing and approving post-graduate training and education is delegated to the postgraduate dental deans. Funding is allocated annually to meet training needs and is based on the number of NHS general dental practitioners, community dental service and personal dental services dentists covered by the deanery. Eligible dentists can claim travel and subsistence for attending Department of Health-funded courses, which includes a meal allowance, night allowance and mileage, where appropriate.

Any NHS general dental practitioner whose name is included on a PCT list or who is a 'Keeping In Touch Scheme' (KITS) member is eligible to attend Department of Health-funded courses. Most of these dentists are entitled to continuing professional development allowance (CPDA) for attending either Department of Health-funded courses or 'other approved courses'. Eligibility to claim this allowance must be confirmed with the dentist's local PCT.

All delegates attending Department of Health approved courses are entitled to an FP84 form at the end of the course. For dentists who are registered with a PCT, this form should be completed accurately and sent directly to their PCT. It is important to retain the yellow copy of the form (whether or not any allowances are being claimed) as this comprises a certificate of attending the course and may be required for future reference:

- in relation to seniority payments
- as evidence required by the Faculty of General Dental Practitioners to support entry to examinations such as Membership of the Faculty of Dental Surgery (MFDS) and Membership of the Faculty of General Dental Practitioners (MFGDP)
- to obtain or retain membership of the Faculty of General Dental Practitioners
- to provide evidence of attendance for recertification/reaccreditation with the GDC.

CPD for community dental services and personal dental services dentists

Dentists working within community dental services and personal dental services contracts may now attend continuing professional education and development courses on the same basis as general dental services dentists and KITS members. They may also access distance learning material previously only available to NHS general dental practitioners and KITS members.

Other approved courses

The postgraduate dental dean may approve the educational content of courses not funded by the Department of Health, known as 'other approved courses'. Approval is granted for specific courses and not for ongoing programmes. The granting of other approved course status indicates specifically that such courses do not attract travelling and subsistence payments.

Retaining and retraining dentists

Loss of confidence, being out of touch with the regulations and lack of knowledge about new techniques and materials are the most common obstacles to returning to dentistry.[5] Dentists are advised to stay on the dental register even if they are away from active practice. The 'Retaining and Returning Adviser' (RRA) initiative was designed to assist dentists to overcome many of the obstacles they face when planning a career break, and to ease the transition back into dentistry.[7]

Keeping in Touch Scheme

The 'Keeping in Touch Scheme' (KITS) was introduced in 1988, and is a national scheme for dentists who have been away from NHS dentistry for at least one year. The dentist must remain on the GDC Dentists' Register, retain membership of a defence organisation and subscribe to a dental journal. In return the scheme:

- pays a contribution towards the dentist's professional expenses
- entitles the dentist to attend approved courses
- entitles the dentist to receive reimbursement of travelling and subsistence for approved courses
- entitles the dentist to obtain CD-ROM distance-learning packages.

At the time of writing the Department of Health funds KITS, but this may change in the future and other funding streams would need to be found, possibly from postgraduate deaneries.

Getting back to practice

Dentists who come off the dental register will have to complete all outstanding CPD before they can reregister. It is relatively easy for dentists to keep up to date and this makes their return to practice easier. Dentists who have been out of practice for a long period will probably need to go on a refresher course. Getting back to practice courses are run in seven centres throughout the UK at different times of the year and are funded by the Department of Health, although future funding may be from postgraduate deaneries.

Summary

The NHS is short of dentists and the cost of undergraduate dental training is high. It is therefore important that there are strategic plans for the recruitment and retention of dentists, and these should include flexible working patterns. In many ways primary care dentistry has been the poor relation of general medical practice, which has an excellent retainer scheme, opportunities for paid returner training and access to prolonged study leave for established GPs. Many of these schemes could be adopted by dentistry if funding was available. There are fewer differences between hospital doctors and dentists because they have the same contracts.

Career counselling is crucial for a significant number of dentists who might otherwise be lost to the profession and it needs to be available for all dentists.

Advice should be given at dental school and available throughout a dentist's career. Mentoring may also be helpful for those dentists who are facing difficulties. Postgraduate deaneries can play a key role in post-qualification career advice, particularly the vocational training adviser and dental tutors.

Further information

- National Centre for Continuing Professional Education of Dentists (www.nccped.co.uk)
- General Dental Council (www.gdc-uk.org)
- British Dental Association (www.bda-dentistry.org)
- Faculty of General Dental Practice (www.rcseng.ac.uk/fgdp)
- MFDS exam information (www.rcseng.ac.uk/fgdp/exams)
- Faculty of Dental Surgery (www.rcseng.ac.uk/fds)
- FDS distance learning course (www.rcseng.ac.uk/fds/distance_learning)
- Evidence-based dentistry (www.cebd.org)
- Cochrane Oral Health Group (www.cochrane-oral.man.ac.uk)
- Dental practice board Dentanet (www.dentanet.org)
- Committee on Vocational Training for England and Wales (www./dvta.org.uk)
- NHS Centre for Reviews and Dissemination (has systematic reviews of research on effectiveness, including filling materials, fluoridation, cancer) (www.york.ac.uk/inst/crd/welcome)
- Bandolier (has enormous range of information on medical (and some dental) treatments; easy to read lively site!) (www.jr2.ox.ac.uk/bandolier/index)

References

1   Morganstein S (1997) Women in dentistry: equal opportunities. *The Dentist.* **13(2)**: 40–41.

2   Seward M (2001) *Better Opportunities for Women Dentists.* Department of Health, London.

3   Department of Health (2001) *Improving Working Lives Standards.* Department of Health, London.

4   Department of Trade and Industry Employment Legislation (2003) *Flexible Working – The Right to Request* (PL516 Rev 1), 6 April, 15.

5   Department of Health (2006) *Primary Care Dental Service: implementation of local commissioning.* Department of Health, London.

6   www.gdc-uk.org/Current+registrant/CPD+requirements

7   London Deanery (2005) *London Deanery Dental Course Guide 05–06.* London Deanery, London.

CHAPTER 5

Flexible working as a consultant

Ian Hastie

Introduction

The National Health Service (NHS) 'Improving Working Lives' initiative[1] makes it clear that there is an expectation that employers should promote a healthy balance between work and life outside work. There is also a wish to encourage flexible working, as this will aid the recruitment and retention of consultants in the NHS. Flexible working has tended to mean working part-time. However, it now has a much wider meaning. Certainly part-time working is still the main group but we are also seeing consultants taking on other responsibilities and changing their work patterns. With the advent of high-speed electronic links through the telephone network and mobile communications consultants do not have to be sitting at their desks. A lot of institutions have internet access to email and some allow access to the institution's computer servers and investigations. This means that consultants can work from home or another site as though they were sitting in their 'office at work'.

In the past most consultants worked full-time or maximum part-time if they had a significant private practice. The demography of consultants is changing and an increasing number, both male and female, are looking to work less than full-time for a variety of reasons, including family commitments, carer responsibilities or mixing clinical work with another career. At the same time, like general practice, there are more and more opportunities for consultants and other career-grade doctors to work less than full-time.

Trusts may not want a full-time consultant as they may be filling a void left by a consultant taking up other programmed activities to work in trust management, within the community or in a postgraduate deanery, etc. Trusts may also not have the monies for a full-time consultant as resources often now come in packages for specific areas of work such as cancer networks and the National Service Frameworks (NSFs).

The old single-consultant firm is disappearing and consultants now often work in multidisciplinary teams, which may include several consultants. This can often lead to consultants not having the same timetable week in and week out. Examples of this include consultants doing a period of time as the acute admitting consultant, with all other duties being cancelled, or if consultants alternate with a colleague a period of time on a ward with a period doing something else, such as research, teaching or outpatients. This can also be planned to fit in with parental commitments such as school holidays.

There has never been a better time for consultants who, for various reasons, do not want to work the traditional hours.

The consultant contract before 2003

The new consultant contract was introduced in England in 2003, for all new consultants and those consultants already in post who opted to change. There were a significant number of consultants who opted to stay with their old contracts and this was often associated with the wish to continue with substantial private practice. Separate contract negotiations were undertaken in other UK countries but the timetable of implementation may not always have been as quick as in England.

The old contract began in 1979, with the basic full-time week estimated to be 11 notional half-days of three and a half hours each. It established three types of contract: full-time (11/11th); maximum part-time (10/11th); and part-time (between 1/11th and 9/11th). The basic difference between the full-time and maximum part-time being that although they both had to fulfil a full NHS commitment, the former was only allowed to earn 10% of their gross NHS earnings privately whereas the latter could earn as much as they wished. The part-timers could work whatever notional half-days were agreed with their employers up to 9/11th of the full-time contract. This allowed them to undertake any other commitment they wished, whether in or out of medicine.

The consultant contract in England after 2003

The new contract was introduced in England in 2003, and applies to all new consultants and those opting to change over from the old contract. The new contract is based on a programmed activity (PA) of four hours' duration (three hours if it is worked 'out-of-hours'). A full-time contract is for 10 PAs, although additional PAs are allowed for extra work. Therefore a consultant, with the agreement of the trust, can work less than 10 PAs per week and be paid accordingly. It is possible, with the agreement of the trust/employer, to have a contract that varies throughout the year. This is particularly helpful for consultants with other commitments which are variable, such as childcare, children's holiday cover or research. The new contract has greatly enhanced the ability to work part-time or flexibly, and often suits not only the consultant but also the trust. The exception to this is that if the consultant is offered an extra PA then that has to be accepted before undertaking private practice. If the request for flexible or part-time working is to carry out private practice, and the consultant was appointed after 1 January 2004, the part-time contract would normally be for six PAs or less, although employers may agree to more than six PAs if they so wish. If the request is mainly for reasons other than private practice the contract can be for more than six PAs.[2]

The contract is made up of two types of PA: those for 'direct clinical care' and 'supporting professional activities'. For a full-time contract these should normally be in the ratio 7.5:2.5. However, as the latter includes areas such as audit, appraisal, clinical governance and personal development, which need to be undertaken by all consultants no matter whether full-time or not, it is recommended that the latter takes on a more significant ratio if working less than full-time. An example would be a consultant working eight PAs: the ratio is recommended to be 5.5:2.5; for a consultant working six PAs the recommended ratio would be 4:2.

Joint jobs

Many consultants now want to work less than full-time as they wish to pursue a commitment outside direct patient care. This may involve a commitment to a managerial or educational role within the trust, a commitment to a university or medical school, a role within the Department of Health or an international agency, a position within a learned society or college, or a position within a postgraduate medical deanery. All of these may make up a full-time contract of varying degrees of commitment to both organisations. Work outside the trust may be undertaken as a separate employment with a specified commitment or may be on a secondment basis whereby the consultant is still employed by the original employer who is reimbursed for the PAs worked outside. In any situation there has to be agreement with all concerned as to what time commitments are involved.

Appointment process

Doctors on the specialist register can apply for consultant positions. Consultant posts are advertised and appointed in open competition, unless there is a statutory exemption. Full-time posts should be available to doctors who want to work less than full-time but the number of PAs has to be mutually agreed and this may not always fit into the needs of the trust. However, more and more trusts are advertising posts that are less than full-time. It may also be that two doctors will apply for a full-time post as a job share.

Academic medicine

The two main areas of academic medicine are teaching and research. Teaching and training is well suited to flexible working, but what about research? It often depends on the type of research that is being undertaken. Clinical research can often be fitted into a flexible work pattern but experimental research, especially if it is laboratory-based, often has tight time schedules and therefore may be less flexible.

Within individual posts there is often a blurred margin between consultant and academic work. Many consultants carry out research in its widest forms and many academics provide clinical consultant service. When both are specifically recognised senior doctors are either paid by the NHS and are consultants with an honorary academic contract, or are paid by the university and are academics with honorary consultant contracts or, rarely now, A plus B with two separate contracts making up the whole. Whatever the contract that the senior doctor holds, since 2003 the time spent on both needs to be clearly defined in the job plan and agreed by all. Difficulties may arise if trying to combine all elements of teaching, research and clinical work within a flexible contract as it may not be possible to give adequate time to all three areas.

Clinical excellence awards

The clinical excellence awards scheme[3] was introduced in 2004 to replace the old distinction awards and the local discretionary points. Recipients have to be NHS consultants or honorary consultants. The new scheme is more transparent, with published criteria for the award. These are equally available to part-time consultants as full-timers. However, the amount of the award is pro rata and dependent on the proportion of full-time work carried out.

Specialist development scheme

In 2005 the Specialist Development Scheme[4] brought together the New Consultant Entry Scheme and the Managed Placement Scheme.

The New Consultant Entry Scheme

This started in 2003 as a pilot offering short-term appointments at consultant level for six months, with the possibility of a further six months if wanted, to specialist registrars (SpRs) who had recently gained their Certificate of Completion of Specialist Training (CCST) and had not yet gained a consultant post. The post would be for a maximum of one year and would not need to go through the usual appointment committee process. As part of the post the Postgraduate Dean would agree a personal development plan (PDP) for the new consultant, which would include a mentor and two sessions for personal development. Employment was through NHS Professionals working in close partnership with the host trust and the usual consultant terms and conditions of service applied. The benefit was that the new consultant had a chance to take on consultant-level work for a trial period before committing to a future substantive post. It gave a structured PDP with support for this first period working in the consultant role. This gave the opportunity to experience working at consultant level in a trust before making a longer-term commitment. For a trust the benefit was that they were able to fill a consultant post for a short term and were therefore able to assess its long-term need.

The Managed Placement Scheme

This scheme provided an opportunity for doctors from overseas to work temporarily as a consultant in, and gain experience of, the NHS. The doctors were initially employed by NHS Professionals, but would be working in a substantive post within a trust, albeit only for up to a six-month period. Following this the doctor could apply in open competition for the post. During the Managed Placement Scheme the doctor would have access to courses on induction to the NHS, regular appraisals and a mentor.

The Specialist Development Scheme

This arrangement brings both schemes together and is aimed at both UK- and overseas-trained doctors. They work for between one month and one year in fixed term placements and each doctor will be assessed to see what level of support is required. The Specialist Development Scheme differs from the two previous schemes in that it brings together the needs of both the doctor and the trust where the placement is taking place.

The Flexible Careers Scheme

The Flexible Careers Scheme (FCS) was introduced as part of the 'Improving Working Lives' initiative introduced by the Department of Health.[1] It aims to enable doctors to have part-time roles and career breaks whilst still keeping abreast of clinical practice and contact with the profession.[5] It allows doctors to change between full- and part- time work, to alter their hours of work, take a break in their career or reduce their work as retirement looms. In addition there are opportunities, after a period of refresher training, to return to work in the NHS.

In particular, it may be of interest to those doctors who want to temporarily reduce their hours, want a career break, are after or coming up to retirement and want to continue working but with reduced hours, want to return to work in the NHS but need a period of supervision, or are presently SpRs who have their CCST and are looking to work up to six PAs as a consultant. (After October 2005 with the commencement of the Postgraduate Medical Education and Training Board (PMETB), the CCST will be replaced by the Certificate of Completion of Training (CCT).)

The scheme is adaptable to the individual and will help with revalidation but is time-limited. Funding is provided from central funds through the deaneries so that for career doctors trusts will receive 50% funding for the first year, 25% for the second and 10% for the third. For returning doctors 100% is paid for six months full-time or one year part-time. In the financial year 2005/2006 the Department of Health devolved the funding for the FCS to strategic health authorities (SHAs) and deaneries, and the budget became cash-limited. This may restrict the opportunities for consultants to join the FCS in the future, unless trusts are prepared to fund in full.

Pensions

Part-time consultants are governed by the same pension rules as full-timers under the new contract. A full-time contract is for 10 PAs, therefore the number of PAs worked as a part-time consultant has to be taken into account. For example, 10 PAs worked for one year by a full-time consultant is equivalent to a part-time consultant working five PAs for two years. For more information see www.nhspa.gov.uk.

Illness/carers/maternity

There are some circumstances in which flexible working is required in the short term. Consultants suffering from sub-acute illness, or during the recovery phase, may wish to work but find that they are unable to work to their normal level. Employers are usually very supportive in these circumstances but individual proposals need to be agreed with the trust. This often involves occupational health staff, who will be concerned about the doctor's capabilities to carry out the work.

Maternity leave is a statutory right under employment law and the terms and conditions of service for doctors, but on return to work doctors may wish to reduce their hours or work to a flexible commitment. This needs to be discussed with the employer because, although they are usually very supportive, it has to be recognised that employers have to provide a service and this needs to be covered.

There are other instances when a doctor may want to work flexibly for a short period of time. It is always better to discuss this with managers, colleagues and the human resources department at an early stage. Since April 2003, as part of general employment legislation, any parent with a child under six years of age or a disabled child under 18 has the right to request to work flexibly and the employer must seriously consider this, although there may be acceptable reasons why it is not possible.

Associate specialist

The associate specialist is a career-grade senior doctor who is responsible to a named consultant. In the past most appointments were on a personal basis but increasingly trusts have advertised for an appointment at this level. The post is usually for a set commitment due to the service requirements. This may be less than full-time and may involve some flexibility, but this needs to be discussed with the prospective employer. Usually these are doctors who are committed to a career in hospital medicine but who do not want to take on the responsibilities of a consultant or who did not complete their specialist training and gain a CCST/CCT and are therefore not on the specialist register. However, with the establishment of the Postgraduate Medical Education and Training Board (PMETB) in October 2005, associate specialists can apply for access to the specialist register following assessment of their previous experience. If successful they are then able to apply for a consultant post in open competition.

The terms and conditions for the associate specialist grade were established in 1991 (HSG(91)18). However, the British Medical Association's Staff and Associate Specialists Committee and NHS Employers are presently discussing new terms and conditions.[6]

Summary

Historically, consultants would be expected to work full-time for the NHS unless they had a private practice or joint academic appointment. The situation has now changed and a substantial number of consultants work flexibly. Initially, this was attributed to the increased numbers of women coming into medicine, but it has been increasingly seen that both male and female consultants want to have a flexible work pattern for a variety of reasons.

It is true, as stated in the Introduction, 'There has never been a better time for consultants, who, for various reasons, do not want to work the traditional hours'. However, with the changing patterns in the workforce this trend will only increase and it will be a challenge to the NHS, as it undergoes change, as to how it can, or cannot, accommodate this need.

Further information

• British Medical Association (BMA) (www.bma.org.uk)

- BMA, guidance on part-time and flexible working (www.bma.org.uk/ap.nsf/Content/CCSCContractpartMS)
- Employment in the NHS, (www.nhsemployers.org)

References

1 www.dh.gov.uk/PolicyAndGuidance/HumanResourcesAndTraining/ ModelEmployer/ImprovingWorkingLives/fs/en

2 British Medical Association/Department of Health (2003) *Part-time and Flexible Working for Consultants*. British Medical Association/Department of Health, London.

3 www.advisorybodies.doh.gov.uk/accea

4 www.nhsprofessionals.nhs.uk

5 www.nhsprofessionals.nhs.uk/doctors/services/flexible-careers-scheme.aspx

6 www.nhsemployers.org/PayAndConditions/non-consultant_career_grade_doctors.asp

CHAPTER 6

New GPs

Clare Etherington and Hazel Richardson

Introduction

Primary care is constantly changing and evolving, and over the past two decades the pace of change has accelerated. There have been two new general practice contracts since 1990, and new frameworks have been set out for the delivery of patient care. Because of a shift from the focus on secondary care, more work is now being done in the primary healthcare setting.

General practice is widely viewed as a family-friendly profession. Doctors no longer join a practice anticipating a 'job for life' so there is much more mobility in the profession, both between posts and between specialties. Opportunities for new general practitioners (GPs) are greater than at any time in the past. There is increasing interest in 'portfolio careers' (combining general practice with other interests) and many more doctors work part-time.

This chapter sets out to look at different flexible working patterns and the training opportunities within them for new GPs, with particular emphasis on higher professional education (HPE) and its past and future challenges, using the experience of the London Deanery as an example.

Opportunities for flexible working

As the percentage of women in the workforce has increased, there has been a demand for more part-time jobs because many of these doctors have to juggle childcare with work. Although it has been possible to work as a part-time assistant, partner or locum, none of these posts carry any inbuilt educational or training component.

In 1972 it was recognised that many women with children were being lost to the profession altogether so the GP Retainer Scheme was started. The guidelines have varied with time, but the principle has been to offer women (or men) with domestic commitments part-time work in a supervised capacity in an approved practice. This meant that these doctors could maintain their skills and confidence until such time as their home circumstances enabled them to return to full-time work. The employing practices had a proportion of the salary reimbursed, thus encouraging them to participate in the scheme.

In 2002 the Flexible Career Scheme (FCS) was introduced, which was available to doctors at any stage of their careers. Again, this scheme fosters part-time working with an inbuilt educational component, but it recognises that some doctors have more complex needs than just the requirement to work part-time. For instance, parents with school-aged children may need to have extra time off work during the school holidays and 'pay back' during term-time.

Other schemes have developed to cover a range of new learners, including GP returners, refugee doctors, EU and overseas GPs. Details of all these schemes can be found on the London Deanery website (www.londondeanery.ac.uk).

Historical background of education for new GPs

The Royal College of General Practitioners (RCGP) recommended in 1965 that GP vocational training should take place over a four-year period,[1] thus emphasising the need for an appropriate length of training with adequate supervision and support to prepare young doctors for the realities of their future working lives in general practice. Despite this, the NHS General Practice Vocational Training Regulations (1979) specified that three years' full-time employment (or part-time equivalent) were required to satisfy the regulations for prescribed experience.

By the early 1990s it had become apparent that GPs were expected to fulfil an expanding role in the NHS and they needed to be adequately equipped for this new kind of job. There had been a change over the years from an apprentice model of training to a more formal structure devoted to the acquisition of a group of core skills. The development of vocational training schemes enhanced this learning process, and the introduction of summative assessment in 1996 formalised it, with appraisal and revalidation producing further change. It was clear that the basic three-year programme of GP vocational training was insufficient for the modern day GP and that there was a need to establish a system of post-vocational training support.

There have been several approaches to this. In 1998 the Committee of General Practice Education Directors (COGPED) published its report on HPE.[2] It was felt that many recently vocationally trained GP registrars would benefit from an additional one or two years of supervision and support in a suitable learning environment. This would increase their preparedness and fitness for their role through a number of approaches, for example:

- enhancing the development of research and teaching skills
- undertaking a masters degree course or similar higher qualification
- developing additional clinical skills

- enhancing information technology and management skills
- generally heightening awareness of the GP's role in the wider primary care context, including the complexities of providing and commissioning care for patients.

The important issue was the need for ongoing educational support at the start of a new GP's career to enhance both competence and confidence. The report noted that although progress was being made in the provision of HPE for new GPs through a variety of educational initiatives in different parts of the UK, there was a lack of a financial framework to make such support generally available. This lack was impeding progress and further development.

The report highlighted various aspects of what was thought to be the appropriate educational context of HPE. These included:

- learner-centredness
- personal learning plans
- the provision of mentoring
- peer group support
- multi-professional or multi-disciplinary working.

In summary it was recognised that newly qualified and returning GPs had learning needs over and above those of established practitioners. With this in mind the concept of HPE was established.

Another report produced in the late 1990s was the final report of the London Initiative Zone Educational Incentive (LIZEI) scheme.[3] This reported on a three-year programme of educational initiatives for general practice from 1995 to 1998. The programme was set within a framework of the four 'Rs', that is Recruitment, Retention, Refreshment and Reflection, and offered many varied training opportunities. The London Academic Training Scheme (LATS)[4] gave an additional period of 12 months of post-vocational training scheme academic training, together with a facilitated support group. Some similar schemes to support new GPs still exist and are sponsored by primary care trusts (PCTs).

The Joint Centre for Education in Medicine also produced an influential report at around this time.[5] This report highlighted the problems of the transition from GP registrar to GP principal, when there is a sudden reduction in educational supervision and support. The report illustrated the reluctance of newly qualified GPs to enter a principal post. It suggested that this cohort of doctors had further training needs and recognised that there was a largely unstructured approach to facilitating further training and development and that, although the vocational training programme might produce GPs competent in terms of basic knowledge and most clinical skills, they might not be 'fit for purpose'.

Health professionals become 'fit for purpose' when they are properly confident and competent to carry out what is regarded as appropriate healthcare provision in the modern setting. For a GP this means:

- having appropriate book knowledge and clinical skills
- knowing how to exercise this knowledge and skill
- knowing how to relate to patients
- knowing how to work in a team
- knowing how to provide services for groups of patients
- knowing how to maintain quality of practice
- knowing how to lay the foundations for life-long learning.

'Fitness for purpose' is a concept that applies equally to individual healthcare professionals (in this case new GPs) and to the healthcare system in which they work. The NHS itself must be fit for the purpose of helping the development of its workforce, in part by providing appropriate opportunities for professional development. As new GPs emerged from their vocational training, it was clear that not being 'fit for purpose' was a real problem. The undergraduate curriculum may not have addressed the factual and life adaptation skills needed to deal with today's healthcare setting and pace of change.

One solution to the perceived training gap was the introduction, in London, of the senior GP registrar (SGPR) scheme in 2000. The purpose was to extend the vocational training period by allowing a further six months' full-time or equivalent part-time supervision in a protected environment. During this period the SGPR was based in a training practice with the associated learning support, and given protected time to develop in additional areas, for example research, teaching, medical specialties. This has now been refined into the clinical fellow scheme, which builds on the strengths of the SGPR project. Posts are self-constructed and combine at least four sessions in general practice with one session of personal professional development, and up to five sessions in other areas working towards the particular needs of the community in which the individual anticipates working. Clinical fellow posts can also be done part-time.

Another solution was the introduction of a national scheme for HPE, and central funding for this came on stream in 2001. Future funding is uncertain but deaneries are keen to continue HPE because of the importance of supporting new GPs.

The strategic importance of higher professional education

As HPE is of strategic importance for the recruitment and retention of competent GPs in the new NHS, the framework for HPE provision had to be designed to withstand at least three clear challenges:

- meeting and supporting the educational needs of new GPs (the transition to independent practice), including constructive help with personal development plans (PDPs) and familiarisation with the appraisal process
- assisting new GPs in becoming fit for the purpose of working in the NHS
- enhancing the retention of new GPs in the GP workforce.

Since government funding for HPE became available on 1 October 2001 it has been managed by directors of postgraduate general practice education (DPGPEs), and deaneries have developed support systems to reach the target group of new GPs. This led to the appointment in London of programme directors to support HPE programmes under the leadership of an associate director of postgraduate general practice education. Various support structures exist in other deaneries.

The evidence that new GPs look for flexible work patterns and initially prefer to engage in roles not requiring geographical or financial commitment is important in planning any supportive provision. Ensuring the 'portability' of HPE support across deanery boundaries adds to its empowering effect. In making individual new GPs feel better supported in their personal and professional development, there are now encouraging signs that retention rates in areas with previously high 'net exporter' profiles, are improving.[6]

Model of HPE delivery within the London Deanery

HPE support is given for two years and is available to all new GPs in whatever capacity they work. The entitlement to HPE is suspended during any career break, for example sickness, maternity leave or travel, and entitlement starts again once work is recommenced. Initially, when funds were plentiful, HPE provided financial support and time out for individuals to pursue personal development agendas. It continues to give a forum for peer support and interactive learning. HPE is delivered on a sector basis in London, with the deanery area being divided into five sectors. Each sector has two programme directors responsible for the HPE doctors on their patch, and for running a locally tailored programme.

The HPE programme directors are appointed and managed by the deanery. They need to be good team workers, communicators and facilitators, have educational and clinical experience in primary care and to establish good relations with vocational training schemes and continuing professional development (CPD), the arrangements for life-long learning for established professionals. They also need support and time to interact with fellow educators with responsibility in this field. The HPE team works closely with others in the London Deanery through a 'GP Educator Development Group'. This stimulates shared learning and exchange of ideas with other colleagues in the deanery educational network The HPE directors in each sector liaise with the local vocational training scheme course organisers and PCT-aligned deanery tutors to ensure that new GPs are aware of the programme. Each new GP is sent a welcome pack and registration form. Once registered, individuals are sent a personal welcome by the sector HPE director and informed about local programmes. Participants are kept aware of events on offer via email cascade. One-to-one meetings allow the director to give practical support in achieving the goals of an individual's PDP.

HPE content

The programme has varied from sector to sector but has usually included residentials, half-day release courses and workshops. The programme directors are also available for further 'one-to-one' support and advice for individual new GPs, and for help with setting up and running self-directed learning groups. In addition to this, all sectors collaborate to run pan-deanery educational events, and programmes are responsive to the needs of HPE doctors.

When new GPs assess their educational needs, it is interesting to see how consistent is the range of subjects raised, with peer support, practice and staff management, change management and information technology heading the list.[7] This reflects the difficulties new GPs face in transition from the closely supported GP registrar post to fully fledged independent practice. Some will seek to develop areas of individual strength, which may contribute to evolving a longer-term locality role such as a practitioner with specialist interest (PwSI). Although a range of educational vehicles has been suggested as a way of optimising HPE delivery,[5] the focus is on encouraging the new GP to move on from the closely supervised model of vocational training scheme day release to a reflective, self directed life-long learning model.

The key features of the programme are:

- Educational support by a programme director in facilitating the planning and execution of individual PDPs.
- An emphasis on self-directed learning groups and peer support to facilitate the learning and development process.
- The provision of a programme of educational events organised by the programme directors and generated by assessment of the learning needs of the group.

Evaluation

An evaluation of HPE experiences so far is being undertaken in the London Deanery, and many of the comments (examples below) demonstrate that the three previously mentioned strategic challenges are being met.

'I think having self-directed learning groups is one of the most important things to encourage GPs, both through funding for groups, assistance in finding a group, and sector half-day releases.'

'Encourages ongoing learning, the creation of a PDP and support from other GPs recently qualified.'

'Makes further reflection on educational needs useful, and urges and enables further education.'

'Helped me start developing my PDP and developing a special interest.'

'Encouraged me to take protected time for self-directed learning. Enabled me to make the most of an excellent learning set by being funded to meet for a session per month, not just an evening after work. Established me in a pattern of life-long learning – thank you very much.'

'As a new principal taking up a partnership direct from VTS [vocational training scheme], I felt there were some huge areas of clinical needs that needed development, e.g. maternity care, consultation skills, specific specialties such as dermatology, intrauterine contraceptive device (IUCD) insertion and chronic disease management, that I wanted to focus on to improve my performance. I would not have been able to get this essential experience to meet my educational needs without HPE. It undoubtedly helped me to survive and improve in my first two years as a GP.'

'HPE was a great scheme. I was lucky enough to be in the right place at the right time to make maximum use/benefit from the scheme. I cannot emphasise enough how important it is to fund this programme adequately. I don't think that it is recognised how difficult it is to progress from VTS to a principal GP without HPE. In London, a difficult and challenging place for GPs, it is definitely a way of retaining good people. Please feed back my appreciation to [the dean, associate dean and programme director] how much the programme helped me to develop as a confident GP and to reduce the stress of the first two years as a principal.'

HPE and modern general practice

Over the last 20 years there has been a dramatic shift in the expectations of both doctors and their patients of how primary care delivery and its associated educational support should function. This generation of new GPs has grown up and entered the profession since the change in GP contractual regulations in

1990, and many are now joining just in time to face the uncharted challenges of the new General Medical Services (nGMS) contract. They often accept that change must occur but are less accepting of how work in general might affect the quality of their personal and family lives. Many GPs are choosing to work part-time or to have portfolio careers.

HPE commenced at a critical time for recruitment and retention. It offers a shield to protect new GPs whilst they develop survival skills. It may increase their confidence as they acquire skills that are relevant to their future practice within the primary care team. The majority of individuals opt for a career in general practice once they have qualified as a doctor.[7] It is therefore important that their experience in the early years of general practice validates their choice.

Support and supervision for the learning and development of new GPs is important as it recognises the value of those individuals to the NHS. It should help to move GPs towards becoming life-long learners and establish a reflective approach to personal development. There has been a cultural shift in attitudes to the role and lifestyle of modern-day GPs. It is now recognised that there needs to be a work–life balance. HPE must ensure that there are appropriate opportunities for self-development and for becoming 'fit for purpose' so that GPs remain committed and enthusiastic about their chosen work.

With *Modernising Medical Careers* (MMC)[8] and the amalgamation of the Joint Committee on Postgraduate training for General Practice (JCPTGP) with the Specialist Training Authority (STA) to form the Postgraduate Medical Education and Training Board (PMETB), medical education has been streamlined so that all doctors have a common foundation before they branch into their chosen speciality. HPE facilitates the transition from new GP to independent practitioner.

Evaluation of the London Deanery and other schemes so far shows how much the programmes are appreciated by the participating doctors. In order to retain the workforce we need to make new GPs feel supported. If new GPs are to be committed to remaining up-to-date and receptive to new ideas and ways of working, a pattern of supported adult learning must be introduced as early as possible. HPE fills this need and should become part of a seamless transition from medical student training through the foundation years and vocational training schemes to the life-long self-directed education programmes of established practitioners; in other words, CPD.

References

1   Royal College of General Practitioners (1965) *Report of a Working Party of Special Vocational Training for General Practice*. RCGP, London.

2   Jackson N and Reiss M (1998) *Higher Professional Education for General Practice: report on current work in the UK based on completed questionnaires from directors of postgraduate general practice*. COGPED, London.

3 NHS Executive (1998) *London Initiative Zone Educational Incentive (LIZEI) Scheme Final Report (Recruitment, Retention, Refreshment and Reflection).* NHS Executive, London.

4 Freeman G (1997) *LATS Second Annual Report 1996-1997.* Imperial College School of Medicine, London.

5 Joint Centre for Education in Medicine (1998) *An Evaluation of Educational Needs and Provision for Doctors within Three Years of Completion of Vocational Training for General Practice.* Joint Centre for Education in Medicine, London.

6 Baron R, Mckinlay D, Martin J, Ward B and Whiteman I (2001) Higher professional education for GPs in the north west of England – feedback from the first three years. *Education for Primary Care.* **12**: 421–429.

7 Bowler I and Jackson N (2002) Experiences and career intentions of general practice registrars in Thames deaneries. *BMJ.* **324**: 464–465.

8 www.mmc.nhs.uk

CHAPTER 7

Part-time partners and sessional GPs

Rebecca Viney

Introduction

Working as a part-time partner or sessional general practitioner (GP) is a route to flexible working in general practice. There are many reasons for wanting to work flexibly, and general practice provides an ideal opportunity for a portfolio career. General practice used to be considered to have a 'flat' career structure, but there are now a wide variety of options that can enhance job satisfaction and keep GPs motivated, including medical education, research, appraisal, primary care trust (PCT) work and clinical work in areas of special interest. GPs should use these opportunities to build a career that best suits them and their individual circumstances.

The annual appraisal is a useful opportunity for GPs to plan their careers, as a match between doctors' careers and their personality is very important. Equally important are personal preferences for the right balance between work and leisure, income, responsibility, type of work and extent of interaction with people. It is also important to recognise that individuals' needs, values and priorities will change with time and need re-evaluating regularly.

What do we mean by flexibility?

Any schedule can be made flexible. Part-time work allows GPs to take on different types of work or spend more time at home. True flexibility, however, includes the use of 'annualised' hours. This means that the total time worked is agreed at the start of the post and this can potentially be changed if mutually agreed. It enables employees to work when it best suits them:

- Example 1: A GP would like to work full-time during term time and take all of the school holidays as leave. On average, this doctor might work 5/9ths of full-time.

- Example 2: A retired GP might wish to travel abroad for extended trips and do extra work in the school holidays when doctors are thin on the ground.

Such flexibility can be achieved by negotiation in any post, or, more simply, by being a locum or joining the Flexible Career Scheme (FCS). The latter also provides good employment terms and conditions, including a strong educational element, although funding for the scheme became cash-limited in 2005/2006. In fact, if mutually agreed, any post could be negotiated to include such flexibility. It is always worth a GP trying to negotiate some flexibility when applying for a post (or soon after being offered a post) and this should be done before signing a contract and starting work.

Primary care organisations (PCOs) and practices in under-doctored areas may be particularly amenable to suggestions of flexibility and a proactive approach is recommended. As GP partners and practice managers find it increasingly hard to recruit, prospective practices are being forced into exploring creative options. There will be pressure on competing practices to provide GPs with an excellent clinical environment, mentoring, career development opportunities and the best contracts.

Drivers for change

The main drivers for change in general practice are:

- The increasing proportion of women doctors (70% of GP registrars are now women).
- Changing social trends towards work–life balance (generation X).
- New national legislation for:
  - equal opportunities
  - disability discrimination
  - flexibility
  - part-time workers.[1]
- The NHS 'Improving Working Lives' initiative.[2]
- The NHS 'Childcare Strategy'.[3]

Over the past 40 years the number of women entering medicine has increased dramatically, and it is predicted that by 2012 women doctors will out number men. In addition, there is a growing desire from both sexes to work flexibly and less than full-time, as part of a wider social trend. For staff working in the NHS this is supported through initiatives such as 'Improving Working Lives'. It is recognised that flexible training is essential and will unequivocally require an increase in the total number of doctors trained.

Specific issues for part-time and flexible posts

In theory the idea of part-time and flexible work is excellent in the quest for personal balance, caring responsibilities, portfolio careers or to enhance job satisfaction. There are, however, some common pitfalls that GPs need to be aware of, as well as some more specific problems for each type of post, which will be described later in this chapter.

Issues common to part-timers

- Time to keep up to date; part-time GPs need the same education as full-time GPs.
- Attending practice meetings is an important part of the job; do GPs attend on their day off or should the practice revolve meeting dates to ensure inclusivity?
- The majority of part-time and flexible posts are salaried, less well paid and not entitled to seniority, although this may be negotiated on an individual basis.
- Sessional GPs are under-represented on local medical committees.
- The contract used is key to job satisfaction: fair terms and conditions enhance job security, self-esteem and quality of life. Partnership and salaried contracts are very variable.
- Appraisal and revalidation will require protected time for preparation, regardless of the number of hours worked.
- General practice is still rooted in the concept that full-time is committed and less than full-time is less than committed.

Solutions for salaried GPs

The new General Medical Services (GMS2) model contract has heralded four new salaried contracts, which have excellent terms and conditions that are roughly the same. The new contracts are:

- salaried GMS2 2004[4]
- salaried PCO employed 2004[5]
- flexible career scheme 2004[6]
- GP retainer scheme 2005.[7]

The General Practitioner Committee (GPC) will publish a model GP Returner Scheme contract in 2005/2006. Unfortunately, there are no national 'model' contracts for practitioners with special interest (PwSI), salaried Personal Medical Services (PMS) GPs or Alternative Provider Medical Services (APMS) GPs.

Therefore GPs are strongly recommended to request that their employer uses the GMS2 salaried contract. Job plans created at the time the contract is signed are invaluable and they protect against imposed changes of workload.

Solutions for practices

- Practices receive some reimbursement via their PCO for the salary of FCS GPs, GP returners and Retainer Scheme GPs, as set out in the Statement of Financial Entitlements for GMS2 practices.[8]
- The new Primary Care Development Scheme[9] could fund flexible posts to improve GP recruitment in under-doctored areas, as funds may be used innovatively by the PCT and allocated to practices or individual GPs.

NHS flexible salaried initiatives for GPs

The GP Retainer Scheme

This scheme was updated in 1998[10] and allows doctors to be employed in an approved practice for up to four sessions per week with educational support, and a small amount of non-GP work may also be undertaken outside the practice. Further details are to be found in Chapter 10.

The GP Flexible Career Scheme

On 29 November 2002 the Department of Health launched the Flexible Career Scheme for GPs.[11] The aim was to provide additional, supported flexible part-time posts for GPs not wishing to work more than 50% of full-time as GPs. It was implemented in response to the recruitment and retention crisis in general practice, the NHS 'Improving Working Lives' standard and new national legislation to provide flexible and family-friendly employment. The scheme aims to demonstrate that part-time flexible working can be a valuable asset to both individual doctors and practices. It enables GPs to strike the right balance between their work and home lives in an educational environment. In this way it helps to support GPs who might otherwise leave the profession because they are unable to find posts that meet their particular needs and it may also encourage GPs who have retired or left general practice to return (*see* Chapter 10). However, in 2005/06 funding for the FCS became cash-limited and this is expected to significantly reduce access to the scheme in future years.

The Golden Hello and the Primary Care Development schemes

In the early 2000s the Golden Hello scheme was used to boost the numbers of GPs in substantive posts, by rewarding them for taking part- or full-time posts with contracts for longer than two years. This scheme ended in April 2005 and was replaced in August 2005 by the Primary Care Development Scheme, which will be used to improve GP recruitment and retention in difficult-to-doctor and deprived locations by offering financial incentives to individuals or practices, and by providing personal and professional development opportunities. Different and innovative ways of using the money are allowed providing it is used for GP recruitment and retention in under-doctored areas. Primary care trusts (PCTs), strategic health authorities (SHAs), local medical committees (LMCs) and deaneries will be expected to work together to ensure the funding is used appropriately.

What is a GP partner?

GP partners were also previously known as 'GP principals'. There are four types of practices:

- the new General Medical Service contract (GMS2) practice
- the Personal Medical Service (PMS) practice
- the PCO-managed practice
- the Alternative Provider of Medical Services (APMS) practice.

All partners are on the PCO 'Provider List' but some partners may not be GPs and are therefore not on the PCO 'GP Performer List'. They might, for example, be the practice manager, the practice nurse or a pharmacist. There are profit-sharing and non-profit-sharing partners. In the author's view, non-profit-sharing partners bear all the responsibility but without the reward. It is strongly recommended that GPs consider non-profit-sharing posts carefully and wisely before leaping into partnership.

The PMS practice

PMS practices were introduced in 1998 to allow GPs to provide more creative posts, and the partners hold contracts as a group with their PCO. PMS practices are paid from an agreed budget providing they meet targets set by their PCT. A PMS practice can recruit a salaried GP when there is a partnership vacancy. However, there is no national salaried PMS contract with minimum terms and conditions, so working conditions are very variable. GPs should ask to see the proposed contract early in the negotiations or better still ask for a quality contract, such as the GMS2 salaried contract, at the start of negotiations. GPs should seek advice over contracts early on from the British Medical Association (BMA).

The GMS2 practice

The GMS2 contract, introduced in 2004, is funded via a number of mechanisms, including the number of patients and Quality and Outcome Framework (QOF) points achieved. The old GMS practice used to lose money if a partner left, as money followed partners. However, GMS2 contract practices are able to be creative with their posts and can choose whether to replace partners with salaried GPs or with new partners. Although the salaried GPs may appear cheaper to employ, the excellence of the GMS2 salaried contract has narrowed the cost gap in some cases. Partners are realising that they cannot push an unlimited amount of work onto salaried GPs as they are contracted to work a finite number of sessions, so if there is a manpower shortfall the partners must soak it up. In addition, the tax rules in the UK make the gross cost of a salaried GP greater than a partner for the same net income.

The APMS practice

There are newly emerging private companies that are taking over the lists of patients where PCTs cannot find suitable GPs to take over the running of practices. These are the new Alternative Providers of Medical Services (APMS). They can employ salaried GPs and other health professionals to provide services for patients.

Advantages of working as a part-time partner

- pay will almost certainly be higher than for an equivalent salaried post
- some practices give equal CPD time for full-time and part-time partners, as a hangover from the Postgraduate Education Allowance (PGEA) of the previous GMS contract, which was equal for full and part-timers
- equal vote in the partnership is usually offered
- the BMA will offer guidance for contract best practice
- entitled to seniority payments.

Disadvantages of working as a part-time partner

- income depends on profits, which can go up or down
- no minimum terms and conditions

- maternity locum cover from the PCT will not cover the actual cost of the maternity leave
- if there is a workforce shortfall partners have responsibility to meet the need, irrespective of their partnership contract
- if the part-time GP has a low superannuable income, no seniority payment is payable under the Statement of Financial Entitlements (SFE); however, there are certain protections for GPs in low-earning practices.

How to organise a fair share of the profits

Many new partners, whether full- or part-time, often find it difficult to understand the implications of being self-employed and no longer having the 'rights' of an employee. In some ways it is like entering a marriage, and requires effort, with give and take on both sides. The partnership contract is a vital legal document that determines the terms and conditions for the partners and should be agreed before joining a partnership.

The partnership is responsible for running the business, so partners will not just be involved in patient care and related administration. They will need to ensure the smooth running and development of the practice as their income depends on the annual profits. Their employees should be suitably paid and their personal development plans (PDPs) supported with appropriate education and training. Most high-earning practices will have loyal and effective staff because the partnership has invested in them. A partnership needs a good practice manager to ensure that the partners do not have to do unnecessary management, although there will always be some management issues the partners will have to be involved with.

When deciding on a fair share of profits the partners need to look at the overall workload of the partners and this may result in a varying amount of clinical work for the same share of profit. For example, one partner may prefer to concentrate on clinical work, while others may be involved in education within the practice, management tasks or outside appointments. This is one of the most difficult concepts for a new partner to grasp but time needs to be allocated for the various activities that should be incorporated into the partners' workloads and may include:

- routine surgeries
- clinics, e.g. baby clinic
- GP with special interest session
- visits
- on-call work
- lead partner for staff development
- lead partner for practice management
- lead partner for information technology

- lead partner for clinical governance
- GP trainer
- educational supervisor
- undergraduate teacher
- course organiser, GP tutor or deanery associate director
- member of the LMC
- PCT appointments
- clinical assistant or hospital practitioner work.

Some activities may not bring in the income that compares to an equivalent amount of time spent on core practice work but there may be knock-on benefits. For example, a GP trainer will have knowledge of good new GPs when the practice is looking for a new partner or salaried GP, and a partner involved with the PCT will understand the relevance of new opportunities for the partnership. Practices have various ways of working out workloads, with some giving points for each activity, whereas others make sure everyone does a proportional share of non-clinical work. New partners may have a reduced share of the profits for the first one or two years while they develop additional skills. New partners may feel this is unfair but many partners look back after a few years and realise that it takes time before they can make a full contribution to the partnership.

Within a partnership there should be the opportunity to increase or decrease workloads and related share of the profits at various points in an individual career. For example, new parents may wish to reduce their workload while their children are small and increase it once the youngest has gone to school or older doctors may wish to reduce workload as they near retirement, or for health reasons.

Some GP partnerships own their premises and the new partner will need to decide whether they want to buy a share. This will usually be offered once they have reached parity and plan to stay in the partnership. Although this may look daunting to a new partner, in most cases owning a share of the premises is to be recommended. The partner will need a mortgage for their share but they will receive a 'cost rent' from their PCO, which can be offset against the mortgage. Any remaining mortgage costs are tax-deductible and the partner should have a good investment as the capital value of the premises increases. Buying a share of the premises should be seen as a long-term investment.

What is a sessional GP?

Sessional GPs were previously known as 'non-principals'. All NHS GPs who see patients must be on a PCO 'GP Performer List' and this includes sessional GPs. Below is a list of some of the many types of GPs contained within this 'sessional GP' category.

- Self-employed (otherwise known as freelance or independent GPs):
    - NHS locum GP
    - agency locum GP
    - out-of-hours locum GP
    - APMS locum GP
    - walk-in centre locum GP.

- Employed (otherwise known as salaried or assistant GPs):
    - salaried PMS GP
    - salaried GMS GP
    - salaried PCT GP
    - salaried APMS GP
    - practitioner with a special interest (PwSI)
    - Flexible Career Scheme GP
    - Retainer Scheme GP
    - Returner Scheme GP
    - out-of-hours GP
    - walk-in centre GP.

Model terms and conditions for salaried GPs employed by both GMS practices and PCOs were published in April 2003 as part of the supporting documentation to the GMS2 contract. The model terms and conditions bring important improvements to the terms and conditions of salaried GPs, in line with the terms and conditions of other salaried doctors in the NHS.[12] The National Health Service (General Medical Services Contracts) Regulations 2004 (Statutory Instrument 2004, number 291) states: 'The contractor shall only offer employment to a general medical practitioner on terms and conditions which are no less favourable than those contained in the Model terms and conditions of service for a salaried general practitioner employed by a GMS practice.'

Specific issues for GPs to consider when seeking flexibility and part-time working as a sessional GP

Locum work

Advantages

- self-employed GP locums can choose their holidays and workloads
- locums can pay into the NHS pension scheme
- the PCT pays for the locum's time to prepare and undertake appraisal.

Disadvantages

- no employment rights relating to maternity, paternity, study leave, annual leave, bank holidays, sick leave, special leave for domestic, personal and family reasons, redundancy
- NHS continuity: after working as a locum for 12 months, continuity of NHS service is lost; this affects future sick pay, maternity and paternity pay
- CPD: no protected time
- revalidation: meeting the criteria for revalidation requires more evidence if a GP is not working in an 'approved system'
- NHS locum pensions: the funding stream for locum pensions may change if employers rather than PCTs have to pay; this will alter the balance and may adversely affect locums
- study leave, annual leave and bank holidays should all be factored into the fees charged by the locum.

Working as a salaried GMS GP

Advantages

- Hours of work, with full-time being defined as 37.5 hours (nine notional sessions of four hours and 10 minutes). Working hours should be carefully defined in a job plan and the ratio of contracted hours in relation to the definition of full-time determines an employee's minimum entitlements to annual leave, public holidays, protected CPD. The salary of part-time employees should be calculated on a pro rata basis; for example, a GP employed for five sessions should receive 5/9ths of the full-time salary for the same job.

- Job plan, which is a key appendix of the GMS2 model contract. This should outline the employee's normal duties, workload and important non-clinical roles undertaken within paid work time, such as participation in practice meetings, clinical governance and primary healthcare team meetings. An element of flexibility between both parties, such as working later when busy and leaving early when not so busy, may be mutually agreed. A brief example of what should be included in the job plan is available on the British Medical Association (BMA) website: 'Focus on Salaried GPs. Guidance for GPs', revised in August 2005, or more fully in the job planning guidance, to be published by the General Practitioners Committee (GPC) in 2005.

- CPD is adjusted on a pro rata basis for part-time workers and is subject to a minimum for Flexible Career Scheme and Retainer Scheme doctors. Full-time salaried GPs are entitled to one session (four hours and 10 minutes) per week on an annualised basis of protected professional development time. The use of the CPD time will depend on the educational needs of the doctor as specified by their appraisal and PDP. The protected CPD time must be used for professional development and it may include time spent developing or updating a PDP, on courses, private study, specific clinical refresher experience and audit. It may also include practitioner group meetings and participation in practice meetings, provided that these have a largely educational component and there is generally sufficient CPD to meet the GP's PDP.

- Appraisal: adequate time must be set aside during working hours for a salaried GP to prepare for the NHS GP appraisal, and additional protected CPD time may be required for this. The GPC has estimated that the first appraisal will require at least 6.25 hours of preparation time, regardless of whether a GP works full- or part-time.

- Maternity, paternity, adoption and sickness benefits: salaried GPs working full- or part-time are entitled to the provisions of the General Whitley Council Handbook. They are entitled to paid and unpaid maternity leave if they have 12 months of continuous service with one or more NHS employers at the beginning of the eleventh week before the expected week of childbirth. For the purposes of calculating whether a salaried GP meets the 12 months of continuous service qualification, the following breaks in service are disregarded (though they do not count as service):
  - break in service of three months or less
  - employment as a GP locum for a period not exceeding 12 months
  - absence due to maternity leave.

In the event that a salaried GP takes leave for maternity, paternity, adoption or sickness leave, the practice will typically employ locums to maintain the level of services that it normally provides. The SFE suggests maximum locum payment to practices, although PCOs have the discretion to pay more, less or none at all. It is recommended that practices should consider purchasing locum insurance to cover their salaried GPs as this would ensure that a practice would be covered in the event of a salaried GP requiring sickness, maternity, paternity, adoption or sickness leave. For further details *see* Chapter 18.

- LMC levies: under the Model GMS2 contract, the employer (i.e. the practice or the PCO) will pay the LMC voluntary levy for the salaried GP.

- Recommended salary: the Doctors' and Dentists' Review Body (DDRB) suggested range for 2005/2006 is £49 248 to £74 816 for full-time salaried GPs (an overall uplift of 3.225% on the 2004/2005 figures). This is only a minimum range and PCO and practice employers have the flexibility to offer enhanced pay rates to aid recruitment, but cannot offer less than this range in assessing the appropriate salary. Personal experience and length of NHS service should be taken into account. The GPC recommends that salaried GPs should ensure that they receive an annual pay uplift in line with inflation and, if available, the government's decision on the pay of GPs following the recommendation of the DDRB. They should also receive an annual pay increment linked to the GP providers' seniority payment scale. The details of this and how it is calculated should be included in the written contract of employment. Salaried GPs add to the quality of services provided by practices and this should be taken into consideration when negotiating salary and future uplifts. Possibilities should be available for salaried GPs to receive a percentage increase or bonus payment on top of their standard annual and incremental uplifts to reflect their contribution to the practice's achievement under the Quality and Outcomes Framework (QOF). Some practices have already committed to reward all their staff with a bonus payment, as they are confident that the practice will gain through QOF.

- Leave entitlements: salaried GPs should be entitled to six weeks' annual leave. Full-time salaried GPs are entitled to 10 statutory and public holidays per annum and pro rata for part-time salaried GPs. This includes two 'NHS days', which NHS staff receive and these two days may be taken at any time by the salaried GP.

- Redundancy: both the GP Retainer Scheme and the Flexible Careers Scheme are for fixed terms. The GPC lawyers have advised that, whilst legally it is generally understood that fixed-term contracts such as flexible careers and retainer schemes can exist, the consequences of having a fixed-term contract and being employed under it for a period of one year or more means that an employee may be entitled to full employment rights. To dismiss a GP because the fixed-term contract (or retainer scheme and flexible careers scheme with funding from the PCO) has come to an end may not be viewed as reasonable and may result in the dismissed employee seeking compensation through an employment tribunal. Employers are obliged to ensure that they have a fair reason for dismissal and that they have followed the correct procedure for dismissal. Obviously, any possible ensuing problems will not materialise should the GP be retained by the practice in an equivalent salaried position. Salaried GPs and their employers are therefore advised to seek individual expert advice from the BMA (if a BMA member) should a problem arise.

Disadvantages

- Seniority payments: the BMA says that salaried GPs should receive seniority payments; however, the practice is not eligible for seniority payments under the SFE for salaried GPs.

- Pay: in general, locums and partners have considerably higher earnings than salaried GMS GPs.

Working as a salaried PMS GP

GPs' experience will predominantly be determined by their contract and the contracts offered are variable, although the BMA advises that those GPs who are employed by PMS practices should receive at least the model GMS2 contract minimum terms.

Working as a salaried APMS GP

Advantages

- Unknown as this is a new type of contract.

Disadvantages

- This will be a growing source of employment but currently there are no examples to evaluate.
- Not NHS employment.
- No NHS continuity for maternity or sickness.
- Does not count towards NHS seniority.
- No model contract.
- No minimum terms and conditions.
- No entitlement to Whitley Council terms of service.

All salaried GPs are strongly advised to join the BMA in order to seek advice before agreeing APMS contracts.

Conclusion

'Doctors who are also mothers with families need to set their own criteria for success and to pace their medical careers over a lifetime, taking advantage of their longevity compared with men! I have seen too many doctor-mothers as unhappy patients because they are simply trying to do too much, all at once. I'm with Robert Louis Stevenson: "It is better to travel hopefully than to arrive, and the success is in the labour." ' (Jill Gordon, Professor of Medical Humanities, University of Sydney)

' "Improving Working Lives" means providing conditions of employment which enable every doctor who wishes to train or work in the NHS to do so to their full potential. My remit, as I see it, is to help publicise to the medical profession and trusts the possibilities for flexible employment and for improving all doctors' working lives. It is also to consider how we might remove the barriers to flexible working. There are many doctors who wish to train and work flexibly – we need them and so need to make this work for them. Trusts have worked hard on IWL for all health workers, but the Department's perception was that doctors had largely been "missed out". So, in conjunction with the intercollegiate committee on Improving Working Lives, the Department of Health suggested the need for a national IWL champion for doctors.' (Eric Waters, Medical Director at the Salisbury Trust)

Further information

- NASGP (National Association of Sessional GPs, previously NANP). Visit the website and join this national association, it has a wealth of information about various types of working. (www.nasgp.org.uk)
- BMA; the general practitioners committee has a sessional GP bulletin – contact jgoodway@bma.org.uk for details.
- Doctors' Support Network (0870 765 0001; www.dsn.org.uk/index.htm).
- www.medicalwomensfederation.org.uk: an independent charity which supports the professional development of women in medicine.

References

1 Department of Trade and Industry (2000) *Part-time Workers Regulations Fact Sheet.* Department of Trade and Industry, London.

2 Department of Health (2000) *Improving Working Lives Standard.* Department of Health, London.

3 Department of Health (2000) *Childcare Strategy.* Department of Health, London. (www.dh.gov.uk/PolicyAndGuidance/HumanResourcesAndTraining/ModelEmployer/ NHSChildcareStrategy/NHSChildcareStrategyArticle/fs/en?CONTENT_ID =4052083&chk=n%2BsSRe)

4 British Medical Association. (2003) *Model Terms and Conditions of Service for a Salaried General Practitioner Employed by a GMS Practice.* BMA, London.

5 British Medical Association (2003) *Model Terms and Conditions of Service for a Salaried General Practitioner Employed by a Primary Care Trust (PCT).* BMA, London. (www.bma.org.uk/ ap.nsf/Content/SalariedGPTCSPCT)

6 British Medical Association (2003) *Model Contract of Employment for a Flexible Career Scheme GP.* BMA, London. (www.bma.org.uk/ap.nsf/Content/flexiblecontract)

7 British Medical Association (2005) *Model GP Retainer Scheme Contract.* BMA, London. (www.bma.org.uk/ap.nsf/Content/contractretainerGP)

8 Department of Health (2004) *GMS Statement of Financial Entitlements for 2004/5.* Department of Health, London. (www.dh.gov.uk/assetRoot/04/06/71/92/04067192.pdf)

9 Department of Health (2005) *Framework for the Primary Care Development Scheme to Replace*

the GP Golden Hello Scheme. Department of Health, London. (www.nhsemployers.org/workforce/workforce-622.cfm)

10 NHS Executive (1998) *GP Retainer Scheme. Health Service Circular 1998/101*. Department of Health, Leeds.

11 Department of Health (2002) *GP Returners and Flexible Career Scheme for GPs*. Department of Health, Leeds.

12 Department of Health (2004) *General Whitley Council Conditions of Service*. Department of Health, London.

CHAPTER 8

Practitioners with a special interest

Imtiaz Gulamali

Introduction

In the process of modernising the National Health Service (NHS) it remains crucial to develop its workforce, and increasing numbers of general practitioners (GPs) want to work flexibly, including part-time. Many GPs have additional skills because some doctors change to a career in general practice after initially training in a hospital specialty, whereas others have acquired specialist skills during their time working in general practice. 'Portfolio careers' have become increasingly popular, in which a doctor has more than one job that might include contracts requiring specialist skills. Developing the role of GPs with an integrated approach to services across the primary and secondary care interface will improve patient access to specialist services in the community, where previously they would have been referred to secondary care. Developing the roles of other primary healthcare staff can also enhance the management of chronic disease in the primary care setting.

The term 'Practitioner with Special Interest' (PwSI) evolved from being called 'Specialist GPs' to 'GPs with Special Interest (GPwSI)' to 'Practitioners with Special Interest'. The term is restricted to mean practitioners with a special clinical interest rather than other interests such as education. The PwSI is first and foremost a generalist, but is also capable of delivering a service beyond the scope of conventional general practice and can receive referrals from other professionals in the primary care setting. The term also includes other professionals, such as nurses, who have developed special interests. This chapter mainly explores the developing PwSI role for GPs and its many ramifications.

What is a general practitioner?

Before attempting to understand what we mean by a GP with a special interest (or PwSI), we need to know what a general practitioner actually is. The definition of a GP varies from time to time as their role changes and develops. However, the latest consensus statement from the World Organization of Family Doctors (WONCA) defines a GP as follows.

> General practitioners/family doctors are specialist physicians trained in the principles of the discipline. They are personal doctors, primarily responsible for the provision of comprehensive and continuing care to every individual seeking medical care irrespective of age, sex, and illness. They care for individuals in the context of their family, their community, and their culture, always respecting the autonomy of their patients. They recognize they will also have a professional responsibility to their community. In negotiating management plans with their patients they integrate physical, psychological, social, cultural and existential factors, utilizing the knowledge and trust engendered by repeated contacts. General practitioners exercise their professional role by promoting health, preventing disease and providing cure, care, or palliation. This is done either directly or through the services of others according to their health needs and resources available within the community they serve, assisting patients where necessary in accessing these services. They must take responsibility for developing and maintaining their skills, personal balance and values as a basis for effective and safe patient care.[1]

General practice is an academic and scientific discipline with its own educational content, research, evidence base and clinical activity. It is a clinical specialty, oriented to primary care, and GPs are specialist physicians trained in the principles of this discipline. A definition of the discipline of general practice must lead directly to the core competencies of general practice. 'Core' competencies means essential to the discipline, irrespective of the healthcare system in which they are applied. The central characteristics that define the discipline relate to abilities that every GP should master. They can be clustered into six core competencies:

- primary care management
- person-centred care
- specific problem-solving skills
- comprehensive approach
- community orientation
- holistic modelling.

To practise the specialty, the competent practitioner implements these competencies in three areas:

- clinical tasks

- communication with patients
- management of the practice.

As a person-centred scientific discipline, three background features should be considered as fundamental:

- *contextual*: usually the context of the person, the family, the community and their culture
- *attitudinal*: based upon the doctor's professional capabilities, values and ethics
- *scientific*: adopting a critical and research-based approach to practice and maintaining this through continuing learning and quality improvement.

The interrelation of core competencies, implementation areas and fundamental features characterise the discipline and underline the complexity of the specialty. Reform of national health systems is a common feature in the UK, as elsewhere in the world. Given the changes in demography, medical advances, health economics and patients' needs and expectations, new ways of providing and delivering healthcare are being sought. It is perceived by policy makers that the traditional models of primary and secondary care are failing to meet the needs of the patients as well as the profession, hence the development of the intermediate-level specialist (the PwSI) to increase access close to the patient while giving support to the wider primary health community.[2]

Historical background to PwSI

Having a 'special interest' is nothing new, and traditionally many GPs have had special interests in subjects such as education, occupational health, management and complementary medicine. Their role in undergraduate and postgraduate education has not only been recognised but adapted in other specialties as well. Take, for example, vocational training in general practice, which is one of the best-evaluated and successful apprentice systems in medicine. Some GPs have taken lead roles in their practices for specific clinical areas centred on general practice tasks, including minor surgery. In recognition of the fact that if GPs offer minor surgery in primary care it results in a quicker and more convenient service for the patient, a financial incentive was incorporated into the 1990 GP contract.[3]

During the period of fundholding GPs were given incentives for providing services not normally considered as core services to their patients, either by themselves or by commissioning secondary care services. Although this resulted in fragmentation and inequity between fundholders and non-fundholders, it did act as a catalyst for GPs to acquire further skills not normally considered as a core function of general practice. It was recognised that a significant number of

GPs were fully competent to perform a wider range of services than were included within general medical services (GMS).

In order to protect and further patient interests, a working group produced guidelines[4] in 1996. The working group was set up by the Department of Health and reported that some GPs had skills to carry out a wider range of tasks than were currently included within their contracts. This led to the production of a set of guidelines whereby health authorities could authorise the provision by GPs of some secondary care services within the primary care setting.[4] Many health authorities approved a few applications, although Bradford Health Authority approved 200 applications and thus became the centre point of research and evaluation.

Fundholding came to an end in 1999 and was replaced by primary care organisations (PCOs), which were initially called 'primary care groups' (PCGs) and later evolved into 'primary care trusts' (PCTs). A cross-sectional survey done in 2001/2002 gave some idea of the numbers of GPs pursuing an outside clinical interest.[5] Although only 40% of the questionnaires sent out were adequately completed and returned, more than 70% of the responders indicated that they had at least one special clinical interest covering over 60 different clinical topics. The vast majority were working as clinical assistants in hospitals, followed by hospital practitioners, with fewer working for their PCG/PCT. In the survey 40% of GPs undertaking special interest work had no contract in place, perhaps undertaking the work in their own practice or privately. The authors of the study concluded that even if none of the non-responders undertook clinical sessions, just by extrapolating the findings of the survey one could assume that there were already 4000 GPs having some special clinical interest outside the realm of traditional general practice. To put it another way, this would mean that even by very conservative estimates nearly 20% of GPs at the time of this survey had some additional special interest.

Obviously this finding raised the question as to what is new about PwSI when we have always had GPs with so-called special interests. It perhaps boils down to giving structure and recognition to their training and work. The key pledge of *The NHS Plan*[6] was to establish 1000 specialist GPs by 2004. In April 2002, the Department of Health and the Royal College of General Practitioners (RCGP) published a paper on implementing a scheme for GPwSI.[7] The paper stated that although the term 'GPwSI' was restricted to GPs, there were many other health professionals, such as nurses, who adopted a similar enhanced role.

In response to *The NHS Plan*[6] the RCGP and the General Practitioners Committee (GPC) of the British Medical Association (BMA) produced their own document,[8] highlighting some of the threats and deficiencies in *The NHS Plan*.[6] The response was critical of the term 'specialist GP' as, in their opinion, GPs are all specialists in family medicine, which they thought was a more demanding clinical discipline than most hospital-based specialties. They were also not in favour of seeing a hierarchical continuum from 'GP' to 'specialist GP' to 'consultant'. They saw each of those roles as equal in their own way, but different. The response also highlighted the importance of making sure that PwSIs are not used as a second-class, cheap alternative to a consultant service. Although there are generally many advantages we should not forget the risks associated with having PwSIs.

The NHS Modernisation Agency has published a step-by-step guide to setting up GPwSI services, which includes how to review current service provision, requirements and service design, clinical governance issues, audit and evaluation.[9] The new GP contract[10] encompasses PwSIs as 'enhanced services' and states that 'these might include more specialised services undertaken by doctors or nurses with special interests' and allows PCOs to commission whatever they consider appropriate for their locality, thereby setting PwSIs firmly within the remit of the PCTs.

Advantages and disadvantages

Before analysing the role of the PwSI, as defined by the Department of Health and the RCGP, we need to look at the threats and opportunities a PwSI service would provide for GPs, patients, academic institutions and the commissioners of clinical services in primary care.

Implications for non-specialists

In response to *The NHS Plan*[6] many universities started training schemes leading to the award of various diplomas. Notable among them was Middlesex University, which offered diploma courses in various subjects such as ENT and diabetes. The first response from the RCGP was that of caution as the then vice-president of the College warned against the culture of 'diplomatosis', which he feared had the potential to undermine generalist medical practice. He said: 'We welcome anything that raises standard for patients, but there is a danger that GPs will feel that if they don't have a diploma in something they won't be able to handle it.'[11] There is therefore a potential for division and conflict within the profession.

Other GPs may be reluctant to refer their patients to fellow GPs, who they consider as generalists like themselves. If patients referred to a PwSI see them in higher esteem than their own GP or decide to re-register with the PwSI's practice it could create further tension within the profession. It is therefore vital that the PwSI role and its remit are clearly set out at the beginning. Involving the local medical committee (LMC) at the initial stage as well as GPs within the locality could avoid these sorts of problems. The other potential source of discontent could come from within the same practice if other GPs are left to compensate for the lost time of their colleague, as working one session as a PwSI is working one session less for traditional general practice. This can only be resolved by having a robust practice agreement and consensus of all within the practice.

There are, however, many advantages, such as easy access and more opportunities for feedback both formal and informal. It could also provide better opportunities for educational interaction between GPs and the PwSIs, in contrast to what generally exists between GPs and consultants. A qualitative study looking at the educational interaction between GPs and hospital specialists found a mismatch between what GPs want from specialists in educational terms and what specialists are providing.[12] It also found that specialists preferred traditional, formal teaching methods but GPs preferred informal, problem-oriented learning. It would therefore be logical to assume that a PwSI would have a better understanding of the educational needs of GPs.

Implications for GPs working as PwSIs

The increasing emphasis on specialisation, even within the same specialty, for example having a cardiologist with an interest in arrhythmias, is considered a natural progression, and general practice cannot remain immune to this trend. Interprofessional boundaries are becoming blurred with allied professionals such as nurses taking on the role of what was considered as traditional general practice.

Professionals like doctors and nurses are taking on new tasks and empowering themselves with new skills, so they can offer services both efficiently and cost-effectively. Such extensions of their role have provided GPs with intellectual stimulation and an opportunity to further their personal development and self-esteem.[13] It can also help prevent 'burn-out' by giving them job satisfaction and variety. The downside is that GPs may become victims of inter- and intraprofessional jealousy, leading to isolation and poor morale. It is important to involve all the stakeholders, including the secondary care sector, in the planning and operational stage of the service.

Lack of support in the form of manpower as well as the proper facilities needed to run an efficient service can also act as demoralising factors, especially if not considered carefully in the planning stage of a new service. We should not forget that the value of generalism might be degraded unless PwSIs practise within their generalist role. The importance of being a good GP first and foremost is of utmost importance. Lastly, bearing in mind the historical background, there is a need to ensure that GPs are not used as a cheap and second-class substitute for a specialist service.

Implications for patients

The implications for patients are summarised as follows:

- patients' needs are met
- choice: not all patients would prefer to see a PwSI in place of a consultant
- better access: ease of access is one of the positives that came out of the evaluation of some of the services run by PwSIs[14]
- shorter waiting times: on evaluating some of the projects, in particular related to PwSIs running ENT services, it became evident that they managed to cut down local waiting lists significantly.[15]

What is not known is the impact of PwSIs on the workload of general practice, also the possible impact on other members of the primary healthcare team and whether it results in longer waiting times to see the GP. There also appear to be gaps in the clinical governance structure, in some cases as highlighted by the director of the Department of Health's clinical governance support team.[16]

Cost implications

There is little doubt that cost-effectiveness is one of the factors behind the whole idea of PwSIs, although, paradoxically, very little is known about it at present. Funding sources for PwSIs are varied and include:

- PCTs
- personal medical services (PMS)
- local development schemes[17]
- earmarked funding for the implementation of a particular national service framework (NSF)
- shifts from secondary to primary care funding (rarely)
- growth funds.

With various sources of funding, it becomes more difficult to analyse the cost critically. To compound the problem further, economic data may not be as generalisable as clinical studies, and different geographical areas will have their unique local histories, interests and contingencies. Efficiency is not the only criterion that directs health service activity, and more important at times is the strength of established interests. A paper looking at the economic perspective of GPwSI services concluded:

> There is currently no evidence to support these changes from the perspective of effectiveness or cost-effectiveness. In many areas GPwSI development will build on existing historical services that may have actually encouraged inefficient use of resources, e.g. the development of minor surgery in primary care may have encouraged treatment of patients who would not have otherwise been treated and who would have made only a minor impact on hospital workload.[17]

Quite apart from the PwSI, we need to look at it from an input versus output perspective:

- **Input (resources)**
  - healthcare professionals
  - medicines
  - premises
  - equipment

- **Output (benefits)**
  - clinical benefits
  - health status and quality of life
  - continuity of care, approachability
  - non-health benefits, e.g. choice, reassurance and accessibility

Implications for monitoring and evaluation

Few of the GPwSI (and now PwSI) services have been evaluated independently. Earlier schemes placed little emphasis on formal accountability and monitoring arrangements, relying instead on professional independence and integrity. More formal arrangements are being developed, including distinct clinical and contractual accountability with regular audit and appraisal. Alongside the assurance of high clinical standards and adherence to established protocols, data need to be systematically collected about outcomes for patients.[18] It is therefore essential that all the seven pillars of clinical governance are considered and put in place before embarking upon any PwSI scheme. These pillars are:

- education and training (including ongoing training)
- workload analysis
- health and safety
- staff development
- patient care
- reflective practice
- audit.

In terms of evaluation, we can consider some of the positive and negative reasons for establishing or not establishing a PwSI service.

- Positive reasons:
  - managing demand
  - improving access
  - reducing waiting time
  - boosting primary care capacity
  - to break the monotony of general practice and help prevent 'burn-out'
  - to help morale and retention in the workforce
  - to compensate for inadequate training at undergraduate and post-graduate levels in certain specialties, such as ENT and dermatology
  - reducing inappropriate referrals to secondary care

- improving the management of workload between the primary and secondary sector
- to help with the education and professional development of GPs.

- Negative reasons:
  - negative impact on an already stretched primary care
  - may create duplication
  - can cause inter- and intraprofessional conflicts
  - creates yet another tier of clinical care
  - lack of evidence of cost-effectiveness
  - lack of proper accreditation in some cases can put both the doctor and patient in a vulnerable position.

To proceed or not to proceed?

Whether a PwSI service becomes an orgy of failure or a shining example of best practice depends as usual on proper assessment prior to setting it up. To help the PCOs, the Department of Health and the RCGP issued guidelines in 2002,[7] which identified the priority areas for PwSIs:

- cardiology
- elderly care
- diabetes
- palliative care and cancer
- mental health, including substance abuse
- dermatology
- musculoskeletal medicine
- women, child and sexual health
- ear, nose and throat
- care for the homeless, asylum seekers and travellers
- other procedures suitable for community settings (endoscopy, cystoscopy, vasectomies, echocardiography, etc.).

This list is not exhaustive as the PCT can develop services in other areas if there is an identified and compelling local need.

How to proceed

- Identify the area for service development.
- The PCT should look at all the options through its commissioning role.
- If a PwSI service is identified as the best option then all relevant stakeholders should be involved, including the acute trust, consultants, patient groups, local GPs, community and social care services.

- The PCT checks if there are guidelines from the Department of Health and incorporates the framework accordingly. Although there are frameworks in place for most of the priority areas, if, for some reason, the specialty chosen is one without a framework, the PCT should contact the Department of Health PwSI National Development Group (NDG), which will delegate the RCGP to develop specialty-specific guidelines after consultation with key stakeholders.
- The contract between the PwSI and the PCT should specify:
  - core activities and competencies required, types of patients suitable for the service, minimum caseload or frequency and reasons for referral
  - the facilities that must be present to deliver that service
  - the clinical governance, accountability and monitoring arrangements, including links with others working in the same clinical area in primary care, at PCT level and in acute trust
  - level of payment.

Before the service can be delivered the following must be in place:

- induction, support and continuing professional development (CPD) arrangements for the GP
- facilities to allow satisfactory delivery of the service
- support of the local population, health professionals and health and social care organisations
- widely disseminated local guidelines on the use of the service
- monitoring and clinical audit arrangements
- appropriate indemnity cover.

Follow up arrangements

When reviewing the service and the PwSI work the following evidence should be sought:

- that the guidelines for the use of the service are being followed
- that the caseload is appropriate
- of relevant CPD, clinical audit, exploration of the view of patients, users and other health professionals, peer observation and revalidation
- of involvement in appropriate clinical governance arrangements, including when appropriate in the local acute NHS trust(s)
- of satisfactory process and outcomes of care, including patient views
- that the generalist service is not being adversely affected.

The PwSI role

Although PwSIs may now be established, the question arises, what are they supposed to do? Three roles have been defined for PwSI by the Department of Health and the RCGP, as follows.

- To deliver clinical care beyond the normal scope of general practice in the form of either an opinion or clinical service on the request of clinical colleagues (e.g. pigmented lesion clinic).
- To deliver a procedure-based service (e.g. endoscopy and colposcopy, etc.).
- To lead in the development of locality services (e.g. lead in diabetes and cancer, etc.).

The type of role a PwSI performs depends upon the specialty, for example a PwSI in ENT may not necessarily be leading the work in the locality, and someone providing a procedure-based service may not provide expert opinion. Even within the same specialty there may be more than one model in existence, as is the case, for example, with ENT.[17]

Skills and training

There appears to be lack of clarity on this issue, as there is no national system for training or accreditation. At present there are two routes for training a PwSI, although there may be a mix of both routes.

- Experiential: the local committees decide the criteria. It is more locally orientated and PwSIs going through this route are less mobile.
- Postgraduate diplomas: usually involving one year part-time training with placements for gaining practical experience. The downside is the cost implications and it may not be oriented to local needs. PwSIs with recognised qualifications, such as diplomas, tend to be more mobile.

Although it is recommended that the PwSI supplements the evidence provided by attending a diploma or similar approved course, there is no requirement at present. In which case, perhaps, the PwSI should have to gain a set of nationally agreed qualifications to iron out inconsistency and protect patients.

The role of deaneries

The role of postgraduate deaneries in supporting PwSIs can be summarised as follows.

- In collaboration with the RCGP making the case for PwSIs and defining the attributes of such a practitioner.

- Contributing to a regional accreditation panel for PwSIs to create uniformity at local and national levels.
- Utilising current deanery education and training programmes or resources to properly support the developing PwSI role. These might include:
  - higher professional education (HPE)
  - prolonged study leave
  - innovative training posts within GP vocational training schemes
  - CPD through appraisal and personal development planning.

Summary

Although the term 'PwSI' is new the concept is not. However, this new term gives recognition to the training and work of many generalist GPs who have pursued other clinical interests. Like any new initiative there is the danger of going down a slippery slope if we lose sight of the original aim and fail to follow the guidelines. PwSIs are generalists with a special interest and not cut-down specialists. As long as they maintain their generalist skills and are trained appropriately for their role, with adequate provisions for their CPD, this can only benefit holistic patient care. It is vital that any intermediate care service utilising a PwSI is well-resourced and developed in tandem with the PCT (or equivalent body) plans after critically analysing all possible options. There is also the need to have a proper clinical governance framework in place. Overall, the benefits of having PwSIs outweigh the risks, based upon the available evidence. This evidence is however patchy and begs further independent research on the subject.

Acknowledgement

This chapter was adapted from:

- Gulamali I and Jackson J (2005) General practitioners with a special interest. In: Hastie A, Hastie I and Jackson N (eds), *Postgraduate Medical Education and Training: a guide for primary and secondary care*. Radcliffe Medical Press, Oxford.

References

1 European Society of General Practice/Family Medicine (2002) *Definition of a General Practitioner: consensus statement on behalf of WONCA Europe*. WONCA, Norway.

2 Williams S, Ryan D and Price D (2002) General practitioners with special clinical interest: a model for improving respiratory disease management. *Br J Gen Pract*. **52**: 838–843.

3 Department of Health (1989) *General Practice in the National Health Service*. HMSO, London.

4   Department of Health (1996) *Health Service Guidelines. HSE (96) 31*. Department of Health, London.

5   Jones R and Bartholomew J (2002) General practitioners with special clinical interests: a cross-sectional survey. *Br J Gen Pract.* **52**: 833–834.

6   Department of Health (2000) *The NHS Plan: a plan for investment, a plan for reform.* HMSO, London.

7   Department of Health and Royal College of General Practitioners (2002) *Implementing a Scheme for General Practitioners with Special Interests.* Department of Health/RCGP, London.

8   Royal College of General Practitioners and General Practitioners Committee of the British Medical Association (2002) *Response to The NHS Plan for England. Intermediate Care and Specialist GPs.* RCGP/BMA, London.

9   NHS Modernisation Agency (2003) *Practitioners with Special Interests. A Step by Step Guide to Setting up a General Practitioner with Special Interest (GPwSI) Service.* NHS Modernisation Agency, London.

10 The NHS Confederation (2003) *New GMS Contract – Investing in General Practice 2003: Section 2.13.* NHS Confederation, London.

11 Royal College of General Practitioners (2001) New round up scheme aims to create 'intermediate' GP specialists. *BMJ.* **322**: 128.

12 Marshall MN (1998) Qualitative study of educational interaction between general practitioners and specialists. *BMJ.* **316**: 442–445.

13 Pringle M (2001) *General Practitioners with Special Interest.* RCGP/RCP, London.

14 Sanderson D (2002) *Evaluation of the GPwSI Pilot Projects within the Action on ENT Programme.* York Health Economics Consortium, University of York, York.

15 Liu HL (2002) Specialist GPs cut ENT wait. *GP Business.* **18**: 40–41.

16 Gerada C (2004) Statement on clinical governance arrangements. *Doctor.* January: 3.

17 Kernick DP (2003) Developing intermediate care provided by general practitioners with a special interest: the economic perspective. *Br J Gen Pract.* **53**: 553–556.

18 Noon A and Leese B (2004) The role of UK general practitioners with special interests: implications for policy and service delivery. *Br J Gen Pract.* **54**: 50–56.

CHAPTER 9

The Flexible Career Scheme in secondary care

Susan La Brooy and Anne Hastie

Introduction

Doctors who have chosen to work in secondary care have found that there has been little choice in the working patterns available, particularly if they aspired to a career as a consultant in a hospital specialty. This is no different from similarly driven people in other careers such as law, advertising and banking. The NHS, when it launched the 'Improving Working Lives' initiative in 2000, acknowledged that changing the culture where working long hours was the benchmark would not only improve recruitment and retention but would result in a happier more effective workforce.[1] Cohort studies in the past have indicated that, although a smaller proportion of doctors in secondary care elected to work part-time compared with general practice, this proportion was not insignificant and was rising.[2,3] A more recent cohort study indicated that the vast majority of female respondents (94%) either currently work less than full-time or may do so in the future, compared with 46% of male doctors in the same cohort.[4]

The Flexible Career Scheme (FCS) was launched by the Department of Health in November 2002 by the Minister of State for Health,[5] and contained retainer and returner options for doctors in training and flexible working patterns for those in career grades. The FCS was intended to expand the options beyond the rather rigid time constraints of flexible training, which requires a commitment of no less than 50% of whole-time working. It has been particularly useful for doctors who wish to maintain their clinical skills while taking a career break, those who wish to return to practice and career-grade doctors who wish to work part-time, either at the beginning or end of their careers.

Doctors who are eligible to join the FCS

- doctors in training grades

- career-grade doctors
- doctors who wish to return to the NHS
- doctors who are not currently substantively employed by the NHS, e.g. locums.

NHS Professionals ran the administration of the FCS until 1 January 2006. The retainer and returner options were quality assured through postgraduate medical deaneries, which assessed and approved application forms. In 2005 the Department of Health decided to devolve the funding for the FCS to strategic health authorities (SHAs) and primary care trusts (PCTs). At the same time the funding became cash-limited, which may affect the future availability of the scheme. However, there is nothing to stop hospital trusts, PCTs and deaneries funding the scheme, where appropriate, as a recruitment and retention tool.

FCS retainer option for doctors in training

The retainer part of the FCS applies to all doctors in accredited training posts, from pre-registration house officer (PRHO), senior house officer (SHO) to specialist registrars (SpR), and will apply to the new foundation programmes and run through specialty training. It includes doctors who are on sick or maternity leave but ceases once doctors have obtained their Certificate of Completion of Training (CCT). The purpose of the scheme is to offer doctors the opportunity to maintain some clinical skills while they take a career break or are unable to work for health reasons. It also offers the opportunity for a more gradual return to work than flexible training, which is required to be at least 50% of full-time working.

Many applicants have used the retainer part of the FCS for family reasons, for example bringing up young children or having to act as a carer for a period of time. These applicants often use the scheme for at least a year, although very few use it for the full two years. Some applicants have also used it to take time-limited career breaks, for sporting events, starting a career in music or other non-medical activities. Lastly, for a few doctors, who have had to stop training for health reasons, it has provided a gradual re-entry to work.

For doctors on the retainer FCS it is important that the maximum time on the scheme (two years) allows immediate re-entry to training. This has been most successful for SpRs who retain their training numbers and therefore retain their training programme posts during their period on the retainer scheme. The majority of the applicants for the scheme have been at SpR level but for PRHOs and SHOs there has been the problem of finding a job in a fiercely competitive field after finishing the FCS. The change of all medical training through *Modernising Medical Careers*[6,7] may make it easier for those in training to use the scheme and re-enter training. However, it begs the question whether doctors who are not in training should also be allowed to access flexible working in the same way.

Application

Before 1 January 2006 an application was made through NHS Professionals, which checked GMC registration and the reasons the doctor was applying for the scheme. The application form together with their curriculum vitae (CV) was then sent for assessment by the local postgraduate medical deanery and the applicant invited for an interview to verify the following:

- the applicant is in a training post
- the reasons and length of time (up to two years) required on the scheme
- whether the type of clinical work and length of time proposed will be appropriate to ensure a return to training
- that the applicant understands the time will not be accredited for training
- that the applicant has discussed re-entry to training with their local clinical tutor or training programme director, if applicable.

From 1 January 2006 individual enquiries about the scheme should be made to the doctor's local postgraduate medical deanery and will be subject to available funding.

Placement

The applicant is responsible for obtaining and organising a supernumerary placement with an educational supervisor for the period of time. A second form is then completed, based on advice from the initial interview and discussions with the clinical tutor or programme director. It must include a job plan and personal learning plan for the period of time requested on the scheme. Most placements concentrate on maintaining specific skills that are compatible with a limited time input, such as outpatients, endoscopy lists or day surgery lists, but the scheme excludes on-call. It is important to ensure that doctors entering the scheme have a re-entry point to training and their experience and time on the retainer FCS allows them to do this. The employing trust is responsible for issuing a contract.

Funding arrangements

- 100% funding for up to two years.
- Maximum 19 hours per week.
- No banding payments applicable.
- Doctor receives £700 per annum towards professional expenses.
- Employing trust receives £1000 per annum pro rata towards study leave expenses.

As funding for the FCS has become cash-limited some deaneries, including the London Deanery, are looking to continue the retainer FCS for doctors in training by using flexible training funding.

Case study

JP, a specialist registrar nearing the end of her training, has always maintained an interest in jazz and was previously a musician. At this point in her career an opportunity presented itself to record her music and get involved in the music business. She took up the retainer FCS for a few months to explore her options and see if her music would be successful. The opportunity was successful and as a result she has gone on to be a part-time consultant and a part-time musician. Without the FCS this doctor may have been lost to medicine (or music).

FCS returner option for hospital doctors who have left the NHS

There is a small but definite loss of trained doctors to the NHS[8] for a variety of reasons, but some wish to return at a later date. Until the introduction of the FCS there had been no defined pathway to return to medicine and the NHS. The returner part of the FCS offers a period of time to refresh clinical skills with a view to re-entering medical practice. This option has only been successful in a limited number of cases, because of the competition for training or career-grade posts once the doctor leaves the scheme. It is most effective where the absence has not been prolonged and expectations of the applicant are realistic. If doctors have been out of medical practice for a long period they need to have limited career objectives, such as a part-time trust doctor post in outpatient diabetic services. It is the career counselling that is critical to the success of returners to medical practice, especially if they have been away for some time.

Eligibility criteria for secondary care returners

The eligibility criteria are strict and the reason for this is to ensure that the short period of refresher training on offer (up to six months' full-time or 12 months' half-time) will enable the doctor subsequently to obtain employment in open competition. Postgraduate medical deaneries have agreed the following criteria:

- all doctors must have full GMC registration
- doctors with restrictions to practice are excluded

- all doctors must have had at least 12 months' employment in a substantive post within the NHS
- all doctors must have been out of clinical practice for no less than two years and no more than five years; if a doctor had been out of practice for more than five years entry to the scheme is at the postgraduate dean's discretion after a satisfactory period of clinical attachment.

Application

Before 1 January 2006 the FCS application form was processed by NHS Professionals, and if it fulfilled the eligibility criteria was passed on to the relevant deanery, with the applicant's CV. The applicant was then interviewed at the deanery to discuss the following.

- Returners' career aims and objectives, to ensure the scheme would be appropriate.
- To suggest the content of their personal learning plan, which should deliver the aims and objectives.
- To suggest the type of placement that would be appropriate.

Doctors wishing to join the FCS after 1 January 2006 should approach their local postgraduate medical deanery. However, placements would be subject to the suitability of the applicant and available funding.

Placement

The majority of FCS returner doctors are placed at SHO level and are given more responsibility as their clinical skills improve. The doctor is responsible for finding a placement and an educational supervisor. A job plan and learning objectives should be agreed and submitted to the dean for approval. The employing trust is responsible for issuing a contract.

Funding

- 100% funding for up to six months' full-time or equivalent part-time.
- Banding payments apply.
- The doctor receives £700 per annum towards professional expenses.
- The trust receives £1000 per annum pro rata towards study leave expenses.

Assessments

Deaneries have had to rely on interviews for doctors wishing to return to training on the secondary care FCS. Where there is concern, a report from a clinical attachment before accepting a doctor to the scheme may be helpful. With the skills and competency assessment tools provided by *Modernising Medical Careers*[9] it should be possible to devise a more objective assessment as an entrance to the scheme and certainly to assess the level of competence on completion.

Case study

AC qualified as a doctor and completed his PRHO year, gaining full registration with the GMC. He then left medicine to train as a minister in the church. Several years later he wanted to return to medicine and train to be a GP so he could combine working in medicine with his work in the church. He obtained a FCS returner placement in care of the elderly and was then successful in gaining a placement on a GP vocational training scheme in open competition. He is currently completing his GP registrar year with view to gaining his CCT.

FCS employment option for career-grade doctors

This part of the FCS seeks to assist career-grade doctors who want to work flexibly for personal reasons or doctors who are semi-retired or approaching retirement. The scheme allows doctors to work up to five programmed activities per week, which can be annualised. The success of retaining career grades in flexible working is a significant proportion of the FCS work and delivers the most in terms of service for the NHS. It deals with people who are already trained and is an inducement to trusts to consider using the medical workforce flexibly in a way that has been long available to other professionals.

Eligibility

- Doctors who are eligible for a career-grade post.
- Doctors who are eligible for non-consultant career-grade posts.
- Doctors who have recently obtained a CCT.
- Doctors in existing career-grade posts.

Funding

The FCS for career-grade doctors offers trusts financial assistance with the doctor's salary over the first three years on a decreasing scale of 50% in year one, 25% in year two and 10% in year three. The trust agrees to a permanent contact and funds the post fully after three years:

- normally funded for a maximum five programmed activities per week
- doctors who have recently acquired their CCT may be eligible for up to eight programmed activities
- any additional locum work must be funded by the trust
- on-call is not included in the scheme
- distinction or clinical excellence awards (CEA) are not funded
- doctor receives £700 per annum towards professional expenses.

Now that the FCS funding is cash-limited this option may have to be funded in full by the trusts in the future, but it remains an excellent tool for retaining experienced medical staff.

Process

Doctors who completed and returned an application form to NHS Professionals before 1 January 2006: if the doctor wants to work in the same trust they should discuss their plans with the clinical tutor and medical director. If the post is in another trust it has to be advertised and the doctor will have to be interviewed in open competition. Deaneries have not been involved in this option of the FCS so there is uncertainty for its future funding, which may have to rely on the employing trust.

Case study

Dr RT was a consultant physician who decided to retire at age 63 years because of the increasing non-clinical work associated with his job. However, he wanted to continue with some clinical work and he joined the FCS. He now works four programmed activities a week doing outpatients, an endoscopy list and ward work. He hopes to continue working until he reaches the age of 70 years.

Appraisal and revalidation

All posts on the FCS should provide sufficient clinical experience for revalidation purposes. Every FCS doctor has a clinical and educational supervisor and his or her post must have a continuing professional development (CPD) element. Annual appraisal should be undertaken in the same way as other career-grade doctors in the employing trust.

Benefits

Doctors on the FCS are entitled to the same range of employment benefits as other NHS employees, such as sickness benefit and maternity rights. Access to the NHS pension scheme is available where appropriate. Benefits for periods of part-time employment are calculated on the whole-time equivalent salary.

Success of the FCS

The number of doctors currently on the secondary care FCS is not high and the majority are in the career-grade option, while the retainer and returner schemes have fewer participants. Most of the retainer FCS doctors have been specialist registrars who have managed a re-entry path to training. It has been difficult to assess the success of the FCS returner option, because the response rate to evaluation questionnaires is poor. In London, of 52 secondary care returners only 10 were successful in obtaining jobs after they completed the scheme.

The future of the FCS

The devolvement and cash limitation of the FCS budget will restrict the use of the scheme unless deaneries and trusts are prepared to give it financial support. If, as predicted, flexible working becomes a reality for the medical workforce, as it already has in nursing, employers will have to respond by offering a range of employment options. This would make it unnecessary to offer financial inducements in the future to trusts for the career-grade part of the scheme.

The retainer and returner FCS may have greater relevance in the range of options that could be offered to doctors as they move through their careers. When all medical training and practice becomes embedded in a skills and competency framework with validated assessments, it will enable objective quality assurance of the FCS, including the competency of doctors as they re-enter practice.

References

1 Department of Health (2000) *Improving Working Lives Standard*. Department of Health, London.

2 Davidson JM, Lambert TW and Goldacre MJ (1998) Career pathways and destinations 18 years on among doctors who qualified in the United Kingdom in 1977: postal questionnaire survey. *BMJ*. **31**: 1425–1428.

3 Lambert TW and Goldacre JM (1998) Career destinations seven years on among doctors who qualified in the United Kingdom in 1988: postal questionnaire survey. *BMJ*. **317**: 1429–1431.

4 British Medical Association (2005) *BMA Cohort Study of 1995 Medical Graduates Tenth Report*. BMA, London.

5 Department of Health (2002) *Flexible Careers Scheme for Hospital Doctors.* Department of Health, Leeds.

6 Department of Health (2003) *Modernising Medical Careers. The Response of the Four UK Health Ministers to the Consultation on Unfinished Business: proposals for reform of the House Officer grade.* Department of Health, London.

7 Department of Health (2004) *MMC; the Next Steps – The Future Shape of Foundation, Specialist and General Practice Training Programmes.* Department of Health, London.

8 Goldacre JM, Lambert TW and Davidson JM (2001) Loss of British-trained doctors from the medical workforce in Great Britain. *Medical Education.* **35**: 337–344.

9 www.mmc.nhs.uk

CHAPTER 10

The GP Flexible Career and Retainer Schemes

Rebecca Viney

Introduction

The GP Flexible Career Scheme and the GP Retainer Scheme are vital schemes to ensure adequate numbers of quality part-time posts. This chapter will explain the two schemes, the differences between them and their advantages and disadvantages.

The original Doctor Retainer Scheme was introduced in 1969. Although the concept was inspired and far ahead of its time, it had severe limitations and only allowed doctors to work two sessions a week in general practice. Education and employment rights were not included. Thus general practitioners (GPs) frequently became deskilled, lost confidence and many never returned to more full-time general practice. In June 1998, the new GP Retainer Scheme was introduced, which includes clinical and educational components with full employment rights. The Department of Health published detailed guidance[1] and the British Medical Association (BMA) produced a model contract.[2]

The Flexible Career Scheme (FCS) was launched in 2002,[3] with an emphasis on flexibility, education and the 'Improving Working Lives' initiative principles.[4] It has made a significant contribution to improving the recruitment and retention of GPs and will facilitate the future uptake of senior roles in primary care by more female GPs. In the financial year 2005/2006 the funding for the FCS became cash-limited, which may limit its future availability.

The GP Retainer Scheme

The new GP Retainer Scheme allows doctors to be employed in an approved practice for up to four sessions per week with educational support and a small amount of non-GP work may also be undertaken outside the practice. The underlying principles of the scheme are outlined in the NHSE HSC 1999/004, which is available to download from the DoH website (www.dh.gov.uk/assetRoot/04/01/19/05/04011905.pdf).

What does the scheme involve?

The scheme aims to facilitate the practice of medicine and career development within a protected and educationally stimulating environment. The post-graduate medical deaneries manage the scheme, and prospective retainees will need to make an application to their deanery.

Who is eligible to join the scheme?

The GP Retainer Scheme is open to all GPs who have a Joint Committee on Post-graduate Training for General Practice (JCPTGP) Certificate[5] or are able to demonstrate acquired rights and intend to return to a career in general practice. From 1 October 2005 the Postgraduate Medical Education and Training Board (PMETB) replaced the JCPTGP, and GPs completing their training after this date will obtain a Certificate of Completion of Training (CCT).

The scheme is not intended for those doctors who are committed to a career in another area, such as GP academics. Usually the retainee will have well-founded personal reasons for undertaking only limited paid employment and the Director of Postgraduate General Practice Education (DPGPE) will take individual circumstances into account when deciding whether to accept a doctor to the scheme.

How many sessions can be worked?

The minimum number of sessions that may be worked per week is one session, and the maximum number of sessions is 52 per quarter, usually spread evenly throughout the period at four sessions per week. On occasion the weekly quota of sessions may be increased to a maximum of six or decreased to a minimum of one, by mutual agreement.

In exceptional circumstances, where a practice cannot offer the retainee the maximum four sessions, the retainee may divide the sessions equally between two separate practices. Prior approval by the deanery will be required for this and it will necessitate the named educational supervisors/clinical supervisors of each practice to liaise and establish good lines of communication.

What additional work can be undertaken?

The retainee may work up to two sessions a week in non-primary care medical services outside the practice with the prior approval of the deanery, for instance as a clinical assistant, out-of-hours work or as a GP tutor. Retainees will also need to notify their defence organisation of any additional work.

What is the duration of the scheme?

The length of time a doctor can be on the GP Retainer Scheme is usually five years, and there is no age limit to joining the scheme providing there is an intention to return to a career in general practice. Retainees are approved to the scheme for a year at a time and must apply annually to be re-approved for their membership of the scheme. Family commitments are by far the most frequent reason given for being on the GP Retainer Scheme and the five-year time limit is very unpopular. Retainees comment that it takes longer than five years before the youngest child reaches school age,[6] but it could also be argued that the five-year time limit does give some protection against producing a long-term ghetto for women GPs. In individual circumstances, and at the discretion of the DPGPE, the scheme may be extended, to a maximum of 10 years (either continuously or intermittently) and maternity leave is not part of this time.

How long is a session?

Under the new General Medical Service (GMS) contract a session is defined as being four hours and 10 minutes. However, if it suits individual circumstances GP retainees may work in fractions of a session, for example three hours or five hours. This includes administrative time and dialogue with the educational supervisor/clinical supervisor at the practice. The retainee may agree to home visits and on-call responsibility, providing this is completed within the agreed sessional time and is in accordance with the educational plan agreed for the retainee with the deanery as well as fitting in with their domestic responsibilities. The sessions of work will be contained in a job plan found in Appendix D of the model GP Retainer Scheme contract.

How does a practice gain approval to employ a GP retainee?

Any practice can be approved for employing a retainee if it can demonstrate that it is working towards core criteria similar to the JCPTGP minimum educational criteria for training practices, over an agreed timescale (*see* 'Modified joint committee criteria' below).

GP Retainer Scheme practice: suitability criteria

GP registrar training practices will meet the criteria for hosting a Retainer Scheme GP, although employment of a retainee will need to be approved by the deanery in order to ensure that the educational element of the scheme is appropriate and the needs of the retainee are met.

Non-training practices may be approved for employing a retainee and will usually be visited by the deanery. The practice should be working towards core criteria similar to the JCPTGP minimum educational criteria for training practices over an agreed timescale.

JCPTGP criteria

- All medical records and hospital correspondence must be filed in practice notes, in date order.
- Records must contain easily discernible drug therapy lists for patients on long-term therapy.
- Eighty per cent summaries in medical records. Practices must be making progress towards these targets. Slow progress in otherwise satisfactory practices should lead to a shorter period of re-selection than the Deanery norm.
- All practices must have methods for monitoring prescribing habits as part of audit, and should have a practice formulary or a prescribing list and a policy on how the list is reviewed and implemented.
- All practices must have a library of books and journals, and internet access at each work terminal.

Educational aspects

- The practice must offer a sufficiently wide range of GMS/PMS services.
- The practice must offer adequate induction.
- The practice must have available help and advice during sessions.
- The practice must make arrangements for the retainee to have a named educational supervisor.
- The practice must notify the deanery of any changes in premises, partnership or employment/educational arrangements of the retained doctor.
- If not a training practice, the educational supervisor should undertake the preparation of the practice and themselves for training and employing a retainee.
- The educational input must be sufficient to meet the needs of the individual retainee and must be guided by a named educational supervisor.

What is the role of the educational supervisor?

A named GP who works regularly within the practice (a performer) should be appointed as the GP retainee's educational supervisor. The rules of the scheme also require that a named clinical supervisor should be available during sessions to provide help and advice, debrief at the end of sessions, and discuss dilemmas and interesting cases if required. In most cases it is found convenient for the same person to fulfil both the educational and clinical supervisor roles. If the educational supervisor is not normally available during the retainee's sessions, the practice must nominate another suitable person as clinical supervisor.

Protected time should be made available for the educational supervisor and GP retainee to meet on a regular basis at a mutually convenient time for tutorial, feedback, case discussion or other aspects of general practice that the retainee feels is needed. A minimum of 20 minutes per week is suggested.

Induction

A good induction is essential. When new GP retainees first join a practice they must go through an adequate induction programme and be provided with a practice information pack. Essential information to include is listed in Appendix B of the BMA's new GP Retainer Scheme contract.

What is the educational component of the scheme?

- Each GP retainee has a practice educational supervisor, whom the GP meets weekly in protected time.
- Each GP retainee submits an annual personal development plan (PDP) to the deanery, which should be locally agreed and dependent upon the needs of the individual GP.
- The GP Retainer Scheme contract contains provision for one session of continuing professional development (CPD) for every eight clinical sessions worked. This provision is in line with the salaried GP contracts within new GMS.
- The GP retainee is therefore entitled to the pro rata full-time equivalent of one protected session per week for CPD. A GP working only one session a week will be entitled to a minimum of eight sessions of CPD per year.
- The GP retainee may be entitled to higher professional education (HPE) where appropriate. HPE (if eligible) is in addition to the GP Retainer Scheme provision for CPD.
- Leave should be taken to attend CPD, or, if it occurs at a time when not normally working, it may be taken as time off in lieu.

Calculating CPD sessions

Based on the new GMS and Retainer Scheme contracts, full-time is defined by clause 4 of the model standard contract terms and conditions:

Full-time general practitioners will normally be contracted to work 37½ hours per working week ('contracted hours'), such hours being divided into nine nominal sessions. Such sessions may be divided up into specific working periods by mutual agreement.

Clause 50 states:

At least four hours per week (pro rata) on an annualised basis shall be protected for activities related to professional development as in the agreed job plan.

Number of CPD sessions per year

- Four sessions per week: 19 sessions CPD per annum.
- Three sessions per week: 15 sessions CPD per annum.
- Two sessions per week: 10 sessions CPD per annum.
- One session per week: eight sessions CPD per annum.

Course costs

GP retainees should approach their practice and/or primary care trust (PCT) for any funding toward the expenses of fulfilling their PDP. PCTs should fund core courses such as resuscitation, child protection and target events, which they have prioritised. Some PCTs have learning accounts for all GPs, including retainees.

Under the Statement of Financial Entitlements (SFE)[7] new GMS practices shall ensure that for any healthcare professional who is:

- performing clinical services under the contract
- employed or engaged to assist in the performance of such services

there are in place arrangements for the purpose of maintaining and updating their skills and knowledge in relation to the services that they are performing or assisting in performing.

Is financial help with professional expenses available?

Under the GP Retainer Scheme, retainees are entitled to a fixed annual sum towards the costs of professional expenses and this is currently (2005/2006) £310. It is paid as a lump sum at the beginning of the scheme and on an annual basis thereafter, whilst the GP remains a member of the Retainer Scheme. Tax and National Insurance are deducted at source, but the allowance is not superannuable.

Defence organisations have a reduced charge for retainees, and for precise up-to-date costs doctors must contact their organisation. Cover for all extra work other than the GP retainer sessions should be discussed and agreed with the medical defence organisation on an individual basis.

What is the payment to the practice?

The practice is reimbursed £59.19 (2005/2006) for each full clinical session and each educational session, as if they were consulting sessions. The reimbursement is intended to offset some of the cost to the practice of employing a GP retainee and supporting them in their educational needs. The practice is also reimbursed £59.19 per session whilst the retainee is on leave, including annual leave, maternity, paternity, adoptive, sickness, an emergency involving a dependent or other pressing family reason.

Contractual issues

Retainees are, by definition, employees. It is a statutory requirement for an employee to have a contract of employment. The BMA's new model contract for the GP Retainer Scheme is in line with the minimum terms and conditions of employment for salaried GMS performers set out in the new GMS contract of April 2004. The GMS employer may not offer employment terms and conditions that are less favourable to those contained in the 'Model terms and conditions of service for a salaried general practitioner employed by a GMS practice'.

Some deaneries, such as the London Deanery, require that any practice employing a GP on the retainer scheme must use the BMA's new model GP Retainer Scheme contract, which must be unchanged. This is to ensure parity and conformity across London for all retainees and avoids a 'post code lottery' of contracts.

How much annual leave can be taken?

Annual leave entitlement is six weeks. It is the intention of the scheme that GP retainees should be allowed to take their holiday entitlement at times that are suitable for their personal circumstances, for example during school holidays, and it should not be a matter of competition with the partners in the practice. The retainee is also entitled to the pro rata full-time equivalent of 10 days bank holidays, which includes NHS days and statutory bank holidays.

What are the maternity/paternity/adoption/ parental leave entitlements?

The Whitley Council handbook[8] currently says:

- *Maternity*: the first eight weeks of absence are paid at full pay, less any Statutory Maternity Pay (SMP) or Maternity Allowance, the next 14 weeks at half of full pay plus any SMP or Maternity Allowance, and the next four weeks at standard rate of SMP.
- *Paternity*: paternity leave is paid at two weeks' full pay.

The Department of Health Advance Letter (GC) 1/2003 is available on the Department of Health website (www.dh.gov.uk/assetRoot/04/06/24/69/ 04062469.PDF). Section 6 of the General Whitley Council handbook explains the maternity leave and pay entitlements of NHS employees under the NHS contractual maternity leave scheme. The contract also allows special leave for domestic, personal and family reasons where doctors are entitled to five days' paid special leave (pro rata).

What sick pay entitlements are there?

Entitlement to sick pay is subject to length of service and is specified in the model contract. It is essential that continuity of NHS service is recognised and agreed before signing the contract.

Tax, NI, superannuation and redundancy

Both the retainee's allowance and retainee's salary are taxable under Schedule E, and the salary of a retainee is liable for Class 1 National Insurance (NI) contributions by the employing practice. All employed sessional GPs are eligible to join the NHS Pension Scheme. In the event a retainee is made redundant he or she will be entitled to redundancy compensation calculated in accordance with Section 45 of the Whitley Council handbook.

The GP Flexible Career Scheme

On 29 November 2002 the Department of Health launched the Flexible Career Scheme (FCS) for GPs.[3] The aim was to provide additional supported, flexible part-time posts for GPs not wishing to work more than 50% of full-time as GPs. It was implemented in response to the recruitment and retention crisis in general practice,[9] the NHS *Improving Working Lives Standard*[4] and new national legislation to provide flexible and family-friendly employment.[10] The scheme aims to demonstrate that part-time working can be a valuable asset to both individual doctors and practices. It enables GPs to strike the right balance between their work and home lives in an educational environment. In this way it helps to support GPs who might otherwise leave the profession because they are unable to find posts that meet their particular needs and it may also encourage GPs who have retired or left general practice to return. Doctors on the FCS work in a substantive capacity.

FCS criteria

The FCS is open to all GPs, regardless of age. It includes the following:

- Those GPs who wish to work 2–5 sessions per week as a salaried GP in an educationally supported post.
- GPs who may want to work part-time in general practice for a variety of reasons, for example they may be a carer, a portfolio GP, an academic, wish to have a career break or downsize near retirement.[11]
- Sessions can be annualised to allow greater flexibility (104–260 sessions per year) to suit doctors' individual needs, enabling doctors to do more work at one time of the year and less at others. For example, parents can take more time off in the school holidays and GPs near retirement may wish to have longer holidays.
- The scheme was initially for four years, providing GPs submitted their application before 1 January 2004 and were in post before 1 April 2004. It was reduced to three years for those applying thereafter.
- GPs submit an application form to their local postgraduate deanery, which determines the eligibility of each applicant to join the FCS and aims to be flexible to individual needs, so long as it remains within the spirit of the scheme.
- Each GP will have a planned exit strategy from the start, which is agreed with the practice educational supervisor and the deanery. This is reviewed annually and the GP is expected to continue with a career in general practice after the scheme expires unless they formally retire. The BMA has advised that all employees with one year of continuous service with their current employer will have acquired full employment rights and may be entitled to compensation for unfair dismissal, including retainees and FCS GPs. Practices can avoid this by retaining the GP in an equivalent salaried position at the end of the scheme. Where possible, it is expected that employers of FCS GPs will make a commitment to their long-term employment once the GP has left the scheme. Where this is not possible, the PCT should work closely with local practices to identify appropriate alternatives.

Other work that can be undertaken while on the scheme

GPs on the FCS are able to undertake additional work, such as educational or clinical assistant sessions, subject to the agreement of the deanery. In 2003 the Department of Health also opened the scheme to locums who wish to continue to undertake freelance work outside of the practice while enjoying the benefits of having a few salaried sessions. The expectation is that where superannuable locum work is undertaken, the equivalent of four or five weekly FCS sessions are worked. Doctors who want to do less than four sessions on the FCS but still do locums must discuss their individual circumstances with their deanery. The deanery exercises its discretion and takes each individual GP's circumstances into account. This extends the reach of the scheme and provides locums with an employment route that enables them access to support for CPD, appraisal, revalidation and clinical governance arrangements.

Approval to employ a FCS GP

Both PCTs and practices can employ FCS GPs. Any practice can be approved for employing a FCS GP providing it can demonstrate that it is working towards core criteria similar to the JCPTGP minimum educational criteria for training practices, over an agreed timescale (*see* earlier 'Modified Joint Committee criteria'). Each practice is individually matched to the FCS GP. Approval of a very experienced GP, for example a retired principal, will need a less rigorous practice assessment than for a relatively inexperienced GP who is working only a couple of sessions per week. As for retainees, postgraduate training practices will automatically meet the criteria for hosting a FCS GP, but employment of a FCS GP will need to be sanctioned by the deanery in order to ensure that the educational component of the scheme is appropriate and generally to protect the needs of the FCS GP. Deaneries must liaise closely with PCTs employing FCS GPs to ensure that any placements are appropriate and that the FCS GP receives the necessary support during any placement with practices.

Educational components of the scheme

These include the educational components for the GP Retainer Scheme. In addition, the practice can claim the full cost of eight sessions of education time (including on-call) for all FCS GPs, irrespective of the number of sessions that they work or number of years in the scheme.

Other benefits of the scheme

The scheme provides the FCS GP with £1050 towards professional expenses such as defence organisations. This is paid by the PCT to the practice and is subject to tax and NI. There is a model BMA contract,[12] which provides terms and conditions no less beneficial than the new General Medical Services salaried contract[13] and reaches the *Improving Working Lives Standards*.[4]

An employer who is committed to improving working lives enables flexibility and:

- recognises the requirement for modern employment in practices
- understands that all staff work best for patients when they strike a healthy balance between work and other aspects of their life outside work
- develops a range of working arrangements, which balance the needs of patients and services with the needs of staff
- values and supports staff
- provides personal and professional development and training opportunities that are accessible to all staff, irrespective of their working patterns
- provides a range of policies and practices that enable staff to manage a healthy balance between work and other commitments outside.

Offering improved working conditions through family-friendly hours in an educationally supportive practice is one of the strategies that a practice can use to attract and retain staff. The flexibility of the scheme can be used as a recruitment tool, enabling practices to be more creative about the way they work. GP partners who wish to reduce their commitment and work more flexibly as they near retirement can convert to the scheme.

A percentage of the total employment costs are met by the PCT on a sliding scale, dependent on the length of time the participant is in the scheme. However, the decision in 2005/2006 to cash-limit the scheme means that funding may not be available for all doctors who wish to join it.

Comparison of the GP Retainer Scheme with the Flexible Career Scheme

Both schemes provide GPs with the opportunity to work both part-time and flexibly in mainstream general practice while balancing their work and personal commitments. However, there are significant differences in the aims of the schemes and in the detail.

- The GP Retainer Scheme is designed to ensure that doctors who can only undertake a small amount of paid professional work (1–4 sessions per week) can keep in touch with general practice, retain their skills and progress their career with a view to returning to a more substantive NHS general practice post in the future. Retainees are re-approved annually and may usually stay on the scheme for five years. The scheme is not intended for those planning a career in academic medicine, portfolio work or other sectors of clinical practice, and they may not undertake locum work. In contrast, the FCS GP is able to undertake additional work as well as their 2–5 sessions on the FCS and can also continue to undertake locum work while employed on the scheme.

- The FCS enjoys job continuity, with a contract for three or four years, and there is an expectation that employers of FCS GPs will make a commitment to their long-term employment once the GP has left the scheme. The BMA advises that all employees with one year's continuous service with their current employer will have acquired full employment rights and may be entitled to compensation for unfair dismissal, including FCS GPs and retainees.

- The GP Retainer Scheme doctor should have well-founded personal, domestic or other reasons for undertaking only limited paid employment and is supernumerary in the practice. In contrast the FCS GP is in a substantive post. This gives the practice an opportunity to include the GP in all aspects of the practice's work.

- The retainee GP may only undertake a limited amount of non-GMS/PMS work, normally no more than two extra sessions per week, whereas the FCS GP may have other employment outside their FCS sessions. The scheme has therefore proved popular with academics, retired GPs, GPs with a special interest in other clinical areas and portfolio GPs. The FCS has also the added benefit of flexibility, which allows GPs to organise their hours around their family or other commitments. In contrast, retainees must work a minimum of one session per week throughout the year, unless on leave.

- The FCS GP's practice agrees to the *Improving Working Lives Standard*[4] and the model FCS contract, which is designed to provide fair employment conditions with similar terms to hospital colleagues as well as the opportunity to have annualised working hours. It has a continuity of service clause, which values and retains these GPs in the workforce. In addition, the practice receives funding towards maternity locums via the PCT. While the Retainer Scheme GPs does not actively include *Improving Working Lives Standard* principals, in practice the new BMA model GP Retainer Scheme contract is almost identical to the BMA FCS contract and provides equally beneficial terms and conditions.

- The retainee GP receives £310 towards professional expenses while the FCS GP receives £1050. Both schemes attract lower medical defence costs due to their membership on the schemes.

The Department of Health has said that the GP Retainer Scheme will continue to operate and complement the FCS, so GPs will have the maximum flexibility in identifying a scheme that best meets their individual needs.

Conclusion

These part-time educational schemes are essential to maintain the flexibility needed to retain the workforce in jobs which have traditionally embraced long hours and a macho working culture leading to much undisclosed ill health, family disharmony, addiction and loss of doctors. Medicine may be the first profession to have made this option available and others may follow its lead. It is hoped that funding restrictions do not lead to the demise of the FCS.

The GP Retainer and Flexible Career schemes are producing a sub-group of doctors working in primary care, but this is not necessarily wrong if the users are happy and the scheme increases the retention of GPs in the current and future workforce. However, various studies[14,15,16,17] suggest that women continue to work part-time in general practice even when their domestic commitments diminish, which has implications for workforce planning.

References

1 NHS Executive (1998) *GP Retainer Scheme. Health Service Circular 1998/101*. Department of Health, Leeds.

2 British Medical Association (2005) *Model GP Retainer Scheme Contract*. BMA, London.

3 Department of Health (2002) *GP Returners and Flexible Career Scheme for GPs*. Department of Health, Leeds.

4 Department of Health (2000) *Improving Working Lives Standard*. Department of Health, London.

5 Joint Committee on Postgraduate Training for General Practice (2004) *A Guide to Certification*. JCPTGP, London.

6 Hastie A (2002) Assessment of the GP Retainer Scheme. *Education for Primary Care*. **13**: 233–238.

7 Department of Health (2004) *GMS Statement of Financial Entitlements for 2004/05*. Department of Health, London.

8 Department of Health (2004) *General Whitley Council Conditions of Service*. Department of Health, London.

9 NHS Executive (2002) *NHS Professionals: flexible organisations, flexible staff. HSC 2001/02*. NHS Executive, Leeds.

10 Department of Trade and Industry; employment legislation (2003) *Flexible Working – the Right to Request (PL516 Rev 1)*. 6 April: 15.

11 NHS Executive (2000) *Flexible Retirement. HSC 2000/022*. NHS Executive, Leeds.

12 British Medical Association (2003) *Model Contract of Employment for a Flexible Career Scheme GP*. BMA, London.

13 British Medical Association (2003) *Model Terms and Conditions of Service for a Salaried General Practitioner Employed by a GMS Practice*. BMA, London.

14 Davidson JM, Lambert TW and Goldacre MJ (1998) Career pathways and destinations 18 years on among doctors who qualified in the United Kingdom in 1977: postal questionnaire survey. *BMJ*. **31**: 1425–1428.

15 Harvey J, Davison H, Winsland J, Seeley S, Ni'Man M and Bichovsky H (1998) *Don't Waste Doctors: a report on wastage, recruitment and retention of doctors in the North West*. NHS Executive, Manchester.

16 Allen I (1998) *Doctors and Their Careers*. Policy Studies Institute, London.

17 Lambert TW and Goldacre JM (1998) Career destinations seven years on among doctors who qualified in the United Kingdom in 1988: postal questionnaire survey. *BMJ*. **317**: 1429–1431.

CHAPTER 11

The GP Returner Scheme

Anne Hastie and Sally Smith

Introduction

Doctors who are qualified general practitioners (GPs) leave the specialty for a variety of reasons, including domestic commitments and other career pathways.[1] Research has shown that 20 years after qualification almost a quarter of doctors are not working in medicine.[2] The recruitment and retention of GPs has become a national priority and *The NHS Plan*[3] required the appointment of an additional 2000 GPs into substantive posts by 2004. One of the most cost effective methods of increasing the number of GPs in the workforce is to recruit doctors who have previously left the specialty.

A number of re-entry courses have been developed in the past with some success.[4,5,6] Baker and Gifford pointed out that future developments such as revalidation would introduce further barriers to re-entry.[7] These authors suggested re-entry training for general practice should be developed further and in a more appropriate and structured fashion.

In November 2002 the Department of Health launched a National Returner Campaign which included the introduction in England of the GP Returner Scheme to facilitate a re-entry programme into general practice through refresher training.[8] The campaign was aimed at qualified GPs in the following circumstances:

- working as locums rather than in substantive NHS posts
- who are not working
- who are working but not in general practice.

The most common reasons for not working in a substantive general practice post are:[1]

- domestic/non-medical work
- working abroad
- pharmaceutical industry

- public health
- other clinical specialties
- GP locum or private GP
- GP Retainer Scheme
- retired.

Application

Doctors interested in returning to general practice apply to their local post-graduate deanery where they are invited for an informal interview to discuss their individual circumstances. Deaneries only had a very small number of doctors returning to general practice each year prior to the introduction of the GP Returner Scheme following which numbers increased tenfold and applications are continuing at a steady pace. It is probable that the increasing emphasis on flexible working has attracted some of these doctors back to the NHS who left because of the previous rigidity of employment within medicine.[9] As a result, many deaneries have developed an infrastructure to assess and support GP returners.

Eligibility

Not all doctors are eligible to join the GP Returner Scheme because of current legislation. The Committee of General Practice Education Directors (COGPED) provided the following guidance on the entry criteria for doctors wishing to join the scheme.

- The doctor must be eligible to work in general practice and evidence should be submitted to the local postgraduate medical deanery.
- They should normally have worked as a GP in the UK or British armed services for at least one year (including as a GP registrar).
- They would not normally be offered refresher training if they had been working in a substantive NHS GP post during the previous 24 months. (There may be circumstances when refresher training is appropriate following shorter periods.)
- The GP returner should normally work at least half-time during the period of refresher training, including clinical and educational activities. Exceptions can be made in individual cases at the discretion of the Director of Postgraduate General Practice Education (DPGPE).
- They must agree to refresh their skills in dealing with GP emergencies.
- They should not work as GP locums during their period of refresher training.
- Returners may work in another field of medicine or in a non-medical career at the discretion of the DPGPE while undergoing refresher training.

- They should indicate their intention to work in a substantive NHS GP post for at least two years (or the equivalent part-time) following their refresher training. This may not necessarily all be completed immediately following refresher training, for example maternity leave.
- Approval to join the GP Returner Scheme is subject to finding a suitable placement.
- Approval is also subject to:
  - full registration with the General Medical Council (GMC)
  - acceptance on to the performer list of their PCT
  - occupational health clearance
  - screening by the Disclosure Services of the Criminal Records Bureau (CRB)
  - medical indemnity
  - clinical references.

A regulatory framework exists, which stipulates those doctors who are eligible to work in general practice. The most recent regulations came into force on 30 January 1998, as a result of the NHS (vocational training for general medical practice) regulations, 1997. Doctors are eligible to work in general practice in the UK[10] in the following circumstances:

- They hold a Joint Committee on Postgraduate Training for General Practice (JCPTGP) certificate of prescribed or equivalent experience.
- They hold a Postgraduate Medical Education Training Board (PMETB) Certificate of Completion of Training (CCT) after 30 September 2005.
- They have a legal exemption to holding a JCPTGP or PMETB certificate.
- They have acquired rights to work in general practice (in some circumstances this only enables the doctor to work as a locum or assistant).

Placement

The GP Returner Scheme allows a period of refresher training of up to six months' full-time or 12 months part-time. This is usually undertaken in a training practice, although the DPGPE can approve placements in other practices with suitable educational support. For most returners it takes between three and nine months from initial contact to the beginning of refresher training for a variety of reasons. It may be difficult to find a placement for some doctors, while others take time before they feel able to make the commitment.

The content of the refresher training, based on a learning needs assessment, varies from one returner to another. For instance, a returner who has been working abroad in general practice may be up to date clinically but need a period of reorientation to the NHS. In contrast, a doctor who has not been working for 10 years because of domestic commitments will need updating in current clinical practice as well as administrative aspects, including the use of information technology in primary care. There have been many changes in primary care over the last decade, with an increasingly multi-professional approach. Exposure to and an understanding of working in a primary healthcare team is particularly important for those doctors who have not worked in general practice for many years.

The GP returner is employed in a similar way to a GP registrar with the practice paying their salary, which is reimbursed by the deanery through their PCT. In addition, the educational supervisor receives the equivalent of a trainer's grant and the returner receives a payment towards their professional expenses (£1050 in 2005/2006).

Assessments

Each deanery will have developed its own system of assessment before accepting a doctor to the scheme. This may include:

- formal interview
- knowledge test, such as multiple choice questionnaire (MCQ) and extended matching questions (EMQs)
- simulated surgery
- self-assessment, including confidence rating scales
- learning needs assessment.

The trainer undertakes regular formative assessments during the placement, tailored to the individual returner, which may include the same tools as they use for their GP registrars.

The COGPED recommends the returner should complete (as a method of formative assessment) at least one and preferably all three of the summative assessment video, written component and MCQ. Summative assessment will be replaced by the new membership of the Royal College of General Practitioners (nMRCGP) assessments in 2007 and will consist of:

- workplace-based assessment
- applied knowledge test
- clinical skills assessment.

Assessments at the end of the placement may include:

- a Structured Trainer's Report or equivalent, which is signed and returned to the DPGPE (or their deanery representative) within one month of the planned finishing date.
- simulated surgery
- exit interview.

It is recognised that some doctors may require rather more rigorous assessment than described in this guidance and trainers should be guided by the DPGPE (or their deanery representative). If difficulties are identified during the period of the refresher training help should be sought from the deanery as soon as possible.

Teaching the GP returner

There are a number of key issues to consider when putting together a teaching package for the GP returner. First, returners by their very nature will come from a variety of backgrounds and will have variable learning needs. Although all returners will have a background of general practice training, they may have been out of practice for many years, on a career break or pursuing another career altogether. Second, it is worth remembering at all times that one of the main aims in teaching is to encourage the development of skills of life-long learning. Involving learners in constructing their individual learning programmes will encourage a sense of ownership and involvement. Third, the learning programme should be fluid and adaptable. Individual needs will change over the period of placement and the teaching must reflect this. For this reason it is convenient to divide the programme into three parts: the first part will cover the core areas that the returner needs to learn or refresh; the middle period will be more variable and may be a good time to consider hot topics, issues arising from day to day practice, and perhaps issues around any assessment requirements. The final period should be based around the exit strategy and preparing for the return to practice.

Learning styles

It would be useful for returners to make an assessment of their preferred learning style early in the programme. This can be done using a validated scale, such as that devised by Honey and Mumford,[11] or more simply by asking returners to reflect on some previous good and poor learning experiences, thinking about what elements gave them a good experience and what that might suggest about the way learners prefers to learn. From this, learners can decide whether their preferred learning style is visual (prefers seeing information, e.g. graphs, pictures), tactile (likes 'hands-on' teaching experiences) or auditory (lectures). Although learners may gravitate towards learning that suits their preference and most will prefer a combination of styles, they should also be encouraged to consider all learning opportunities. It is useful to bear in mind the preferred learning style when considering learning activities in the personal development plan (PDP).

Educational tools

Returners should be encouraged to develop their PDP at an early stage. The process of doing this will encourage reflection and the learning activities planned will feed into the learning programme. The educational supervisor and the returner can use the PDP as well as a variety of other tools to construct the individual teaching programme. These tools could include the returner's curriculum vitae (CV), self-assessment using MCQs and rating scales, video consultations, the returner's reflective diary, and consideration of local and national requirements. Returners will have had an opportunity for self-assessment with an adviser from the deanery prior to placement and the findings of this will help inform the teaching. Clearly, the teaching programme will evolve over a period of weeks and will change throughout the placement as new needs arise. Using the division into core, middle and final stages, as suggested earlier, will provide form and structure.

As well as encouraging returners to keep a reflective diary throughout the entire placement, which will help inform the learning programme, returners should also keep a record of 'PUNs' and 'DENs'. This is a useful scheme devised by Richard Eve.[12] PUNs are 'patient's unmet needs' and DENs are 'doctor's educational needs'. Numerous PUNs and DENs can be identified in every surgery and Eve suggests documenting them, identifying the need arising and planning how the need will be met. Some of these identified PUNs and DENs can be incorporated into the PDP. Along with their CV and the outcome of their initial deanery assessment, returners will now have several tools which can be used to construct their PDP, and from this, their learning programme.

An example of the PDP might look something like Table 11.1.

Table 11.1: An example personal development plan

Identified learning need	How identified?	Planned activity	Intended outcome
Need to be able to do computer searches for project	Not able to extract data from computer	Training with practice manager	Completion of project
Understanding osteoporosis	PUN	BMJ learning module	Better understanding and explanation to patient

It is best to limit the PDP to five or six learning activities as more than this may become unmanageable. As with the actual teaching programme, the PDP will also evolve during the refresher training placement.

Learning programme

The initial part of the teaching programme will probably be the most structured. Having considered the initial assessment, the returner's CV and learning needs arising from that, along with core topics such as consultation skills, basic practice management and current issues within general practice (e.g. quality assessment), it will be possible to plan a teaching programme individualised to the returner. Using a variety of teaching methods and encouraging returners to be involved in the planning as well as leading some sessions will help to encourage returners to use the skills of life-long learning. The middle section of the training programme is likely to address some of the issues arising from formative assessments as well as allowing discussion of current issues and problems arising from consultations. The final section of the learning programme will be variable in length, as it will depend on the issues that have previously arisen. It would be helpful at this stage to spend some time reflecting on the placement and the learning programme and perhaps carrying out further self-assessments in order to ensure that the identified learning needs have been fully addressed. It is essential to leave enough time for this stage so that topics can be revisited if necessary.

Returners will have spent time within an educational environment during the placement and it is worth spending some time towards the end of the placement encouraging them to think about personal strategies to ensure that they continue to be able to access educational opportunities. The educational supervisor should be aware of local educational opportunities, such as postgraduate educational meetings, self-directed learning groups (SDLGs) and, if appropriate, higher professional education (HPE). They should be able to help returners to make initial contacts with the GP tutor, the local SDLG leads and HPE programme director. Returners may also value the educational supervisor's advice and local knowledge when looking for a suitable job.

Educational supervisor

Educational supervisors are usually, but not always, approved GP trainers. However, they must have appropriate experience of teaching and training. Educational supervisors should not feel solely responsible for providing tutorials for every teaching session. Although returners should have protected learning time, this may involve self-directed study or sitting in with other professionals, including members of the primary healthcare team and consultant colleagues, as well as tutorials with the educational supervisor. Clearly, the educational supervisor has a valuable and crucial role in helping returners to get the most out of their placement by ensuring the teaching is individualised to returners' particular needs and by encouraging returners to develop the skills of life-long learning. A successful placement will be invaluable in ensuring the smooth return of these crucial members of the general practice workforce of the future.

Exit strategy

The initial interview with the individual returner prior to placement should identify an exit strategy, which may need to involve the local PCT. The refresher training needs to take into account the type of employment doctors are planning for their future. If they want to work exclusively as a salaried GP assistant they may not need to include practice administration, but this would be important for someone hoping to become a partner in a practice. Peer support for returners is important and the deanery is in a position to co-ordinate a peer support network. At the end of the period of refresher training the doctor may require further support and this can be provided through various activities, including mentoring and self-directed learning groups.

An exit interview with the DPGPE or their representative is helpful and gives the deanery feedback on the GP Returner Scheme, with suggestions for improvement. In addition, the interviewer should discuss with returners their future career intentions, educational needs and other issues. Comments for those who have already finished the scheme have been overwhelmingly positive and include:[1]

'Confidence boosting'
'Supported in what I wanted to do'
'Getting back to work in a protected environment'
'Excellent resources and information about the scheme'
'Equipped to move back into general practice'
'Support was there when I needed it'

One GP returner who completed and benefited from the scheme wrote about his experience so it could be shared with future applicants.

The GP is privileged. Always an adviser, occasionally an expert, frequently an educator, often a confidante, sometimes a friend, of necessity a counsellor and, if lucky, a mentor. So, it was with some trepidation that after 14 years of having left the NHS, and not having seen a patient in that time, I decided I wanted to practise medicine again.

Why trepidation? Many reasons given the duration of my absence, and changes in UK medical practice over the years. I had issues around knowledge, confidence, skills, information technology, protocol and bureaucracy. I was neither sure of myself nor of my ability.

But I was lucky.

Under the auspices of the London Deanery, I was taken under the wing of a supervising trainer and into a quality general practice. I was gently re-introduced into the processes of primary care, and re-educated accordingly.

Via direct training in the consulting room, supervised and videotaped consultations, regular tutorials, participation in practice meetings, attendance at VTS meetings and 'homework', I regained my 'emotional composure' and my clinical expertise.

Six months on, I am a productive, valuable contributor to the UK healthcare system once again.

I would highly recommend the GP Returner Scheme to anyone.

Summary

The GP Returner Scheme has been an important and successful initiative to increase the recruitment of GPs. The scheme has been particularly useful as a means of helping women doctors return to general practice after a period of not working due to family commitments. The total cost to the Department of Health for a GP to undertake the maximum six months full-time on the scheme in London is approximately £50 000, which is considerably less than the cost of three years' vocational training to produce a new GP.

References

1 Hastie A and Clark R (2005) The GP Returner Scheme: the London Deanery experience of the first 50 applicants. *Work Based Learning in Primary Care.* **3**: 23–30.

2 Goldacre MJ, Lambert TW and Davidson JM (2001) Loss of British-trained doctors from the medical workforce in Great Britain. *Medical Education.* **35**: 337–344.

3 Secretary of State for Health (2000) *The NHS Plan: a plan for investment, a plan for reform.* Department of Health, London.

4 Baker M, Williams J and Petchey R (1997) Putting principals back into practice: an evaluation of a re-entry course for vocationally trained doctors. *Br J Gen Pract.* **47**: 819–822.

5 Stephens C (2000) The participation of women returners to general practice in a re-entry course: another lost tribe? *Br J Gen Pract.* **50**: 730–731.

6 Muller EJ (2002) How we teach on a 'Return to General Practice' course. *Medical Teacher.* **24**: 590–593.

7 Baker M and Gifford B (1998) Returning doctors to medicine. *BMJ.* **316**: 2–4.

8 National Health Service (2002) *General Practitioners – Returning to the NHS.* Department of Health, London.

9 Vaughan C (1995) Career choices for Generation *X*. Young doctors want flexible career paths, not long term commitments. *BMJ.* **311**: 525–526.

10 Joint Committee on Postgraduate General Practice Training for General Practice (2002) *A Guide to Certification.* JCPTGP, London.

11 Honey P and Mumford A (1986) How to choose learning activities to suit your style. In: *Using your Learning Styles*. Peter Honey Publications, Maidenhead.

12 Eve, R (2000). Learning with PUNs and DENs: a method for determining educational needs and the evaluation of its use in primary care. *Education for General Practice*. **11**: 73–79.

CHAPTER 12

Academic medicine and dentistry

Leanda Kroll and Jane Roberts

Introduction

There are still very real barriers to part-time working in some fields. For example, in universities it is almost impossible to find anyone in a senior position who is not working full-time, and often doing 60–70 hours per week. Within the field of clinical academic medicine in particular, there is no culture of part-time working or of training in a part-time post, as the pressures of combining clinical work, research and teaching are felt to make it impossible.[1]

This chapter hopes to present an optimistic yet realistic account of the current state of clinical academia and the possibilities for flexible training and working within it. Although much of the evidence presented relates to academic medicine, the issues are very similar in academic dentistry, which is in an even more perilous state.

Academic medicine and dentistry are not enjoying a 'golden age'. Extensive media coverage often links these terms to the phrase 'in crisis' and there have been dramatic calls for 'resuscitation'.[2] Doctors or dentists contemplating a career in academia might be forgiven for thinking that this is not the most propitious moment to commit themselves to a professional life of scholarly pursuit.

Traditionally, clinical academia has been viewed as comprising three core areas: research, teaching and clinical work. A fourth pillar draws the three areas together in seeing a scholar as able to integrate and apply knowledge from all three domains, culminating in improved healthcare for patients.[3] This is a tall order. Most clinicians would be hard-pressed to maintain competence and job satisfaction in any two out of these three activities. As this chapter will later discuss, although medicine remains an inherently traditional profession, a climate of change is occurring and the 'feminisation of medicine'[4] and dentistry, that is, the increased proportion of women entering the workforce, is leading to challenge of the status quo.

The crisis in academic medicine and dentistry

So what is the crisis in academic medicine and dentistry? The term refers to the diminishing number of academic posts across all grades. Each year the Council of Heads of Medical Schools (CHMS) and the Council of Heads and Deans of Dental Schools (CHDDS) report on clinical academic staffing levels. The 2005 report[5] makes for depressing reading in parts:

> Whilst clinical academic numbers in medicine have remained stable at the most senior levels, numbers of clinical lecturers have declined a further 17%. In dentistry, numbers of clinical academics have actually declined in all clinical academic grades from the lowest levels in a decade seen in 2003.

Academic medicine is an ageing profession. With the further loss of clinical lecturers 'there is an inexorable decline in the traditional seedcorn of academic medicine'.[5]

> A number of academic medical specialties are currently in a perilous position; four specialties (pathology, anaesthesia, psychiatry and radiology) are currently operating with fewer than 75% of the numbers returned in 2000, in pathology this is just 44%. The same is true of many of the dental specialties. The nation needs good quality clinical academics in all specialties. Failure to support them will
>
> - compromise patient care
> - threaten the UK's position as a world leader in medical research
> - remove our ability to educate the doctors and dentists of the future.[5]

The most recent CHMS survey confirms the trend:

> A detailed survey this year shows a further reduction of 14% in lecturer posts in 2004 underlining the deep-seated crises in academic medicine. This is despite four new medical schools coming on stream, and a 40% increase in medical student numbers in the last few years.[6]

The loss of doctors from academia has largely been into the National Health Service (NHS) with its security of contracts, transparent career structure and greater financial remuneration. This is particularly true for women who 'are five times more likely to leave the academic work force at an earlier point in their careers than men'.[7] One consultant had considered an academic career but had abandoned the idea. She had done a PhD at a prestigious teaching hospital and could have gone on to a senior lectureship, but had settled for a consultant post elsewhere: 'I decided I would not be able to juggle everything – to be a good clinician, plus do the research, plus have a social life and a family life. I couldn't do a senior lecturer job part-time. I'd get kicked out.'[8]

Education and research in medicine and dentistry in the UK is highly regarded internationally and yet an academic career is not perceived as attractive.[7]

Challenges and issues: setting the scene

In December 2003, the British Medical Association (BMA) produced a report entitled *Encouraging Women to Work in Academic Medicine*,[7] which serves as a useful benchmark when reviewing the current picture of academic medicine in the UK. The report also identifies that many more doctors of both sexes are keen to work flexibly. This observation is supported by the tenth report of a BMA study of 1995 medical graduates.[9] Recognising and addressing gender issues is an essential part of the current debate and redressing the gender dimensions of academic medicine, specifically in the areas of student selection, curriculum content and career progression for academic staff[10] will have a positive impact on human resources and healthcare for everybody – patients and staff alike. Reichenbach and Brown[10] state emphatically: 'We believe that the goal is not just ensuring equal numbers of men and women (gender equality) but also guaranteeing fairness and justice in the professional opportunity structure (gender equity).'

The authors of this chapter support the pursuit of gender equity and, whilst it may appear to be written for women (particularly the discussion of obstacles), addressing the gender inequity which currently exists will benefit all those doctors who wish to experience a healthier work–life balance.

Medical schools are sustained by the excessive effort of committed individuals to teaching, research and clinical activity. Working long hours and not stepping off the treadmill is a choice that can no longer be the expectation for clinical scientists of any age or sex.[7]

What are the current issues in academic medicine?

- Serious difficulties in recruitment, especially at junior levels, although here the numbers of women are relatively higher.
- Loss of women from academic medicine at every stage of the hierarchy.
- The expectation of excessively long hours for what has traditionally been seen

as 'two jobs in one', precludes those doctors who wish to have healthy personal lives.
- The paucity of positive role-models at senior levels.
- Women have been marginalised within academic medicine with respect to salaries, awards, resources and space.[7]
- Measures of success centre on competition for and performance in research funding, with other important but competing demands on clinical academics' time (including teaching) undervalued.
- Flexible working patterns are seen as 'less productive'.

How has this situation arisen?

The present structure of academic medicine has developed, in parallel to other specialties, within the long-established traditional culture of medicine. The term 'culture' is much contested within social science disciplines, but for the purpose of this discussion refers to 'a set of shared understandings, beliefs and practices' which, in medicine, have gone unchallenged until relatively recently.

Medicine has long been viewed as a highly traditional profession which has rarely welcomed change and has maintained a 'rigid and conservative career structure'.[8] Its inflexibility particularly jeopardises those doctors whose career routes are unorthodox or 'M-shaped':[8] the so-called 'peak, dip and peak' distribution, the 'dip' often occurring during child-rearing years. The 2004 BMA report, *Women in Academic Medicine: Challenges and Issues*[11] illustrates this aspect of career progression, often seen in the narratives of women's careers. The report contrasts this with the 'single trajectory' approach that most 'successful' (usually male) careers have taken.

> Most women have a tortuous career path, they come from a different angle, it's not the main stream, it's looked at as a handicap instead of being looked at as an advantage, because these people have got so much commitment that they went through all these hurdles to do what others are doing as a straight line. Why people can't see that this is an advantage, these women are so motivated to keep going, despite all the obstacles they keep going, they never give up.[11]

Other elements of the traditional culture of medicine which have fostered its current expression include the heavy reliance on sponsorship and patronage, which underpins much of recruitment and promotional practice. Many groups of doctors have been disadvantaged by this system, notably doctors from ethnic minorities, those who have trained abroad, doctors working less-than-full-time and women doctors (with or without children). A system of patronage that rewards and promotes on the basis of personal connections and disregards measures of competence is totally unjustifiable, as well as being likely to flout legal recommendations for equal opportunities and anti-discrimination practice.[12] This climate will not, however, change overnight and many doctors, in particular those who have strongly benefited from the status quo, are resistant to change.

The flipside to a culture of patronage is the presence of bullying,[13,14] which has long existed and gone unchecked, particularly where doctors have not had access to supportive mentors and where promotion depends on job references from those who may have been complicit with the intimidating behaviour.

Finally, an implicit 'ageism' has existed whereby doctors are expected to have reached certain milestones in their career trajectories by a certain age with no allowance made for doctors who have career breaks. This has indirectly hampered career development for many women.[11]

> There has been some belated recognition that the straight full-time career path so engrained in the mindset of the medical hierarchy could be open to change. But suspicion remains of those who have more unconventional career paths or who have not reached a certain grade by a certain age.[8]

The future

As previously indicated, the status quo is being challenged by the feminisation of medicine and also by the BMA through the Medical Academic Staff Committee (MASC).[6,15] A series of new initiatives, combined with a desire to tackle the crisis and improve the structure of academic medicine, potentially herald a new era. An enthusiastic clinician scientist, Rebecca Fitzgerald, summarised both the attractions and the obstacles of a career in academic medicine: 'For people with a passion for the intellectual challenge of research with added opportunities for teaching and international travel, an academic career should be very attractive.'[16]

However, she acknowledges the practical problems that have impeded many trainees:

(1) Lack of a clear career structure.
(2) Insufficient flexibility to be able to combine doctoral research training and clinical training.
(3) Prolonged insecurity about the length of tenure and the financial rewards.[16]

Seeking solutions to these substantial obstacles has fallen under the remit of the NHS *Modernising Medical Careers* (MMC) committee, which has seized the opportunity to look critically at academic medical training programmes. At the same time the government has made extra money available for research and development (R&D) and created the UK Clinical Research Collaboration

(UKCRC) 'to harness the power of partnership between government, industry and medical charities in order to establish the NHS as the world leader in contributions to clinical research.'[17] The UKCRC provided an umbrella under which to bring together the Department of Health, the NHS and those medical charities responsible for training and employing clinical academics. The joint sub-committee of the UKCRC and the MMC, chaired by Dr Mark Walport, (Director of The Wellcome Trust) produced an important report, colloquially known as 'The Walport Report'.[17]

The Walport Report

In addition to the deterrents to a clinical academic career previously described, the Walport report also noted the lack of a clear route of entry and the paucity of geographical mobility in the current system. A shortage of properly structured and supported posts on completion of training was also identified as a potential problem. The report concluded with a statement of key recommendations. The crux of the proposals centres on the needs of trainees rather than employers and on a multi-level approach, which addresses the four stages of a clinician's career (*see* below). The core proposal comes during specialist training with the introduction of dedicated academic training programmes in medicine and dentistry in partnership with local NHS trusts and deaneries.

Stage 1: medical school

The report recommends that students are taught by inspiring clinical academics and informed of academic medicine as a career option. Opportunities exist during the special/selected study modules (SSM) and throughout the curriculum. An intercalated Bachelor of Science (BSc) should be encouraged and supported and Bachelor of Medicine/Doctor of Philosophy (MB/PhD) programmes, which combine undergraduate training with research, should be funded and participants followed up, although no procedure is outlined. It is suggested that similar opportunities for higher degrees should be developed within medical education.

Stage 2: foundation programmes

There are three options proposed, depending on the previous academic interest and experience of trainees.

- For those who have demonstrated a strong interest, such as MB/PhD students, a pilot two-year integrated academic foundation programme, providing clinical and academic competencies but with a reduced clinical time commitment.

- For those who show 'an aptitude and commitment for a research/educational career', an integrated Foundation Year 2 (F2) programme in one academic department, which encompasses academic activities throughout the year, including access to an academic mentor, attendance at academic departmental meetings, project work and a taught component.
- A four-month academic rotation within F2; a 'taster' option.

Stage 3: specialist training

This is the core proposal of the report (*see* Figure 12.1). It recommends that dedicated academic training programmes be developed, consisting of two phases:

- Phase 1 'academic': the academic clinical fellowship phase (a new development) with an academic national training number (NTN (A)) leading to a competitive externally funded training fellowship. Clinical posts will take place within a strong academic environment; however, only 25% of the time can be spent on academic pursuits, with service demands proportionately reduced. The training will last a maximum of three years. Two hundred and fifty fellowships will be offered each year. If the fellows want to pursue further research full-time, they would normally apply for a training fellowship (*see* below) to complete a higher degree over a further three-year period.
- Phase 2 'clinical': the clinical lectureship phase, leading to the certificate of completion of training (CCT) after completion of a higher degree. Funds awarded will allow 50% of time to be spent on academic activity and are allocated to individuals not institutions, allowing geographical flexibility.

For an interim period it is proposed that 100 new clinical lecturer posts are introduced each year by national competition for those currently completing training fellowships, until the first academic clinical fellows finish Phase 1.

Trainees will receive joint academic and clinical appraisal throughout phases 1 and 2, and can return to a solely clinical training route at any time, subject to satisfactory outcomes. Although offered as the primary route to an academic career, the report concludes that other entry points should still be accepted, although these may be relatively poorer in terms of limiting competencies and thereby competitiveness. An equivalent scheme is proposed for medical educationalists (*see* Figure 12.1).

A dedicated academic training programme is also recommended for academic dentistry, which mirrors the scheme outlined for medicine at all stages.[17]

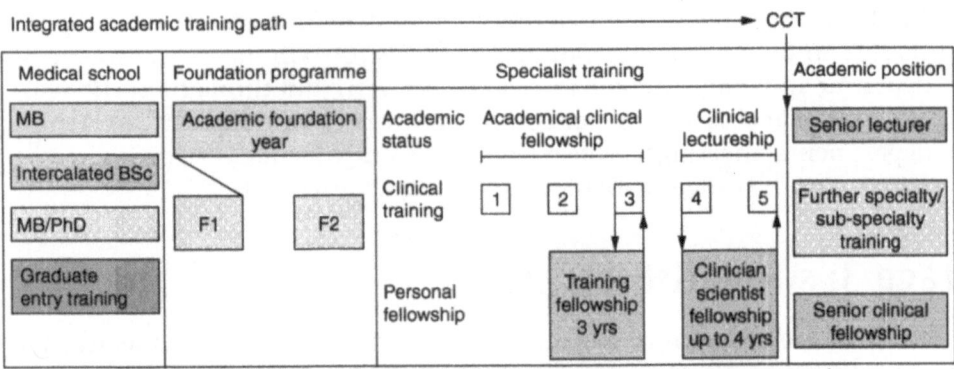

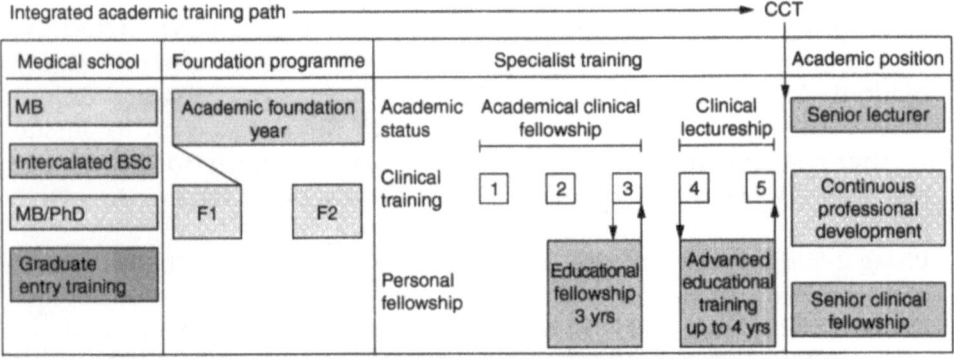

Figure 12.1 Training pathways for researchers and educationalists.

Stage 4: post-certificate completion training

A cohort of 'new blood senior lectureships' is proposed for academic medicine and dentistry to accommodate the new generation of trained clinical academics exiting the proposed training programmes at consultant or senior academic GP grades, and to help them establish their careers. They should be funded jointly by the NHS and universities or medical charities, and assured of pay parity with their NHS counterparts. A clear route back to clinical medicine, supported by additional training if necessary, should also be provided. NHS and university partners will facilitate this if there is clear joint 'ownership' of academic staff.

No new recommendations have been made for PhD fellowships, which remain the core of academic training. All are subject to individual application, although clearly requiring the support of a reputable and high research assessment exercise (RAE) ranking institution.

A range of possible schemes for training fellowships exist, and these include the major donor institutions:

- NHS research and development awards exist at three levels: doctoral, post-doctoral and career scientist, and these offer an option of training at 70% full-time equivalent (FTE) (four years at 70% compared to three years' full-time training).[18]
- The Wellcome Trust has three levels of fellowship, including an entry to doctoral studies with research training fellowships for clinicians (which recognises time out for maternity leave); intermediate and senior research fellowships.[19]
- The Medical Research Council, which offers clinical fellowships.[20]

Recommendations for general practice

A key principle of the Walport report was to consider general practice as equivalent to other specialties and avoid awarding it 'special status', which can lead to marginalisation. On completion of Foundation Year 1 (F1), graduates may apply for a restricted number of F2 placements. Funding for these posts will be provided by the deaneries, and approximately 5% of all placements in F2 will be academic placements, some as academic GPs. After the recommendations from the Walport report, two options for entry into academic general practice are planned.

Academic vocational training schemes

This option involves completion of a three-year vocational training scheme (VTS) with the addition of a further 12 months divided between service and academic training, according to the nature of the bid. These schemes are integrated into the new vision of academic medicine and will be part of the total 250 new allocations. Applications will be submitted centrally as a joint bid between the postgraduate deanery, university and local NHS trust for national competitive selection. Schemes will then recruit candidates locally using existing structures.

Post-vocational training scheme academic training in general practice

This route proposes a 12-month full-time equivalent (FTE) post, which is likely to be carried out in parallel with clinical work with a probable 50:50 split over two years. Doctors would be responsible for arranging their own clinical placement, supervision and funding, which would be linked and may well come from the workforce development directorates (WDDs) or local trusts. The National Coordinating Centre would fund the academic element for research capacity development, awarded on the basis of a successful competitive application, with a well-defined content, which might include a master's degree. These schemes will be awarded on the same principles as the academic vocational training schemes with joint bids made between universities deaneries and the local NHS trust.

The Walport report and family-friendly working practices

Although no specific recommendations were made in the Walport report for flexible training or working less than full-time, the committee considers that applications will be made on an individual basis and expression of interest in working less than full-time should be considered favourably. However, the report acknowledges the particular challenges which arise with career breaks, in a gender-neutral section entitled 'Family-friendly working practices':

> While clinical academic medicine will always be challenging and competitive, there is no reason why family-friendly working practices should not be encouraged.[17]

The report proposes carefully structured support programmes and additional mentoring before and after a career break. It recognises the deskilling that can occur during prolonged absences and suggests that academic mentors plan ahead for the break and keep in touch with and help update mentees during their absence. In addition, there should be 're-entry programmes', to reintroduce mentees to the research environment upon their return, and opportunities to 'brush up' clinical skills.

The significance of the Walport reort

As with clinical training, wherever there is a clear structure with flexibility there is the possibility of training flexibly by working fewer sessions per week and prolonging the overall time period for training. The Walport report, in discussing the need to recruit and retain more women, notes 'while gender parity seems to be attained at the training fellowship level, this is not the case at postdoctoral and senior level'.[17] At present only 20% of doctors doing training fellowships go on to academic careers.[15]

Since women reach their late twenties and early thirties at the training fellowship stage, they need to be aware of their 'biological clocks'.[21] In a changing culture, funding bodies and higher education institutions need to provide additional support and opportunities for flexible training and working. Walport has provided the template to do this for all academics:

> It is not just about modifying the expectations of an academic career to encourage wider participation by women. Today's doctors are rejecting the demands and lack of support by senior colleagues and instead are lobbying for improved working conditions, promotion, better equity and less hierarchy in the workplace. There has been a change in attitudes to work by both genders.[7]

The research assessment exercise

The strains of the present system for research assessment are problematic for all staff, but women are especially hard hit when it comes to establishing and maintaining a research career.[7]

The research assessment exercise is the means by which the quality and quantity of research produced in UK higher education institutes is assessed within given parameters. How 'productive' researchers are and whether their work is submitted are critical issues, since funding is awarded per capita included in the research assessment exercise submission of the higher education institute. The research assessment exercise is sponsored by the four UK funding bodies for higher education and, depending on the outcome (or 'quality profile'), each higher education institute can expect more or less funding for its future research staff and administration.

Depending on the subject, expert panels are configured and sent in to examine and assess 'research outputs', 'research environment' and 'esteem'. There are two main panels set up to cover medical subjects (A and B), whilst C covers dentistry. Higher education institutes are asked to divide their various research departments into groupings of related subjects or 'units of assessment', which are then rated. Pre-clinical and human biological sciences, for example, might be chosen as a unit of assessment.

In the consultation document for research assessment exercise 2008[22] the largest weighting (75%) for 'research quality' will go to 'research outputs' (publications, ideally in 'high impact journals') with four publications expected over seven years. A proposed 20% of the weighting is to be attributed to the 'research environment,' which includes numbers of PhD students under supervision, research training, research income, strategy and infrastructure. Lastly, 5% of the weighting will go to 'esteem', which includes committee membership of funding bodies, editorships of major research journals and, for young researchers, competitive fellowships or prestigious awards.

Criticisms of the research assessment exercise

There are many criticisms[23] but those relevant to this chapter concern the exclusion of certain groups from the previous research assessment exercise (2001), 'in proportional terms, males were 1.9 times more likely to be counted as research active'.[24]

Women who had had career breaks (many academic grants do not have provision for maternity leave) and those working less than full-time were often considered 'less productive' and not included in the submission:

> Women are less likely to apply for research funding, in part due to their under-representation in senior grades, or by being on a fixed-term contract, which makes them ineligible for some grants. They are less likely than men to be involved in a range of high profile academic activities, to have a high publication record (affecting RAE scores) and a PhD.

The 2004 BMA report[11] was based on two focus groups of women at various stages in their academic careers. One aspect of academic medicine that caused concern for many participants was gaining recognition for publications, and many felt that there was discrimination against them as women, both directly and indirectly. In part, this was attributed to collaborative research not being acknowledged or rewarded, with only first authors gaining credit. In other cases, career breaks, less than full-time work and a tendency to 'multi-task' meant that many women were not seen to be as research active as their male colleagues.[11] The BMA report recommended research output should be linked to hours worked:

> Forms of assessment and accountability, such as the RAE, must be made more flexible in order to take into account part-time and flexible working arrangements and career breaks and measure output in terms of achievement, not hours worked. A RAE target of 60% research output for part-time academics is suggested as a measure of addressing this issue. The teaching aspect of an academic career must also be taken into account and valued more explicitly.[11]

The structure of the previous research assessment exercise in 2001 led to higher education institutes making 'strategic' decisions not only with regard to which researchers would be submitted but also the organisation of their departments. This included the 'sudden' acquisition of 'world class researchers' (and their track records) on the eve of the research assessment exercise, dramatically boosting the subsequent rating. At the other extreme, respondents to a recent BMA survey on the research assessment exercise 2008[23] were aware of the dismissal or forced resignation of 'non-productive' staff and of bullying and harassment of staff seen as not performing to research assessment exercise standards. In addition, the research assessment exercise paid no credit to excellence in clinical practice or in teaching, a weakness of the system which has had devastating consequences to some institutions and individuals.

During the 2005 annual presentation to the BMA, Professor Michael Rees, Chair of Medical Academic Staff Committee (MASC), was forthright in his condemnation of the iniquitous practices that have arisen in response to the criteria of the research assessment exercise:

> The main cause of this crisis [decrease in academic posts] is the way institutions have responded to the pressures of the research assessment exercise (RAE). MASC has already highlighted the loss of many university science departments as a result of the RAE. The education of medical students is a clear strategic need. This cannot be subject to a free market RAE approach as the country needs a defined supply of doctors. The RAE has devalued the role of education and resulted in the destruction of many clinical academic departments needed to teach students.[6]

A better research assessment exercise in 2008?

The current review of research assessment for the research assessment exercise 2008[25] incorporates a number of changes which may be helpful. Since 2004 a consultation process has considered modifying the research assessment exercise in response to the criticisms that have been levied against it. The review cycle has been extended to seven years (four publications expected) recognising the long-term nature of research.

In an important shift of emphasis, instead of an overall rating for each unit of assessment, a 'quality profile' is produced showing the percentage of research activity in the submission judged to meet the standard for the appropriate star rating[15] and staff are not individually rated. Thus 'pockets of excellence' can be identified, and there is no disincentive to include all eligible staff. In fact, there is clear encouragement to include 'all excellent researchers' in 2008,[15] not least because of important changes in equal opportunities legislation since the last research assessment exercise.[12]

There is guidance for higher education institutes from the Equality Challenge Unit and an equality briefing for panel chairs, members and secretaries.[12] The legal constraints upon the research assessment exercise focus upon a higher education institute's submission decision with regard to demographic variables of age, disability, race and gender. All higher education institute submissions have to be 'defensible' in respect of equal opportunities legislation, and universities will be encouraged to present their decision-making processes as transparent and fair. An additional caveat concerns the status of staff on fixed-term and part-time contracts, who now have the right to be treated comparably with 'permanent' employees. We need to be mindful, however, that new laws may have little immediate impact on established practices and we may not see any demonstrable change in the 'old culture' for a long time.

With regard to encouraging a new culture, the research assessment exercise process at each university is expected to foster professional development:

> Departments should describe the arrangements for developing and supporting staff in their research, including how this support sits with their non-research duties. Departments should submit evidence of how their policies have had a positive outcome in supporting the career development of young researchers, clinical academics and category C staff [the latter are not employed by the higher education institute but are independent investigators active in research] and for integrating them into a wider supportive research culture.[22]

The demands of clinical work and training are also recognised as 'mitigating circumstances'. NHS academic staff and junior academics (pre-CCT) may submit only two publications. This qualification also applies to dentists and to those 'clinical academics with substantial clinical commitments' in academic general practice.[22] 'This measure is intended to encourage the maintenance of clinical research environments involving research-active NHS staff.'[22]

It seems odd in this consultation document to describe the clinical workload of a clinical academic as a 'mitigating circumstance', although it might be seen to be an improvement on the previous situation where research was expected to be conducted in one's spare time. Other, more conventional mitigating circumstances have also been listed, which signals a positive move towards a more humane and just research assessment exercise. These include working less than full-time, post-maternity/adoptive leave, chronic disability (if diagnosed after October 2006), absence through ill health or injury and new entrants to the profession (regardless of age). These are welcome modifications and, again, signal a positive change in the structure and culture of academic medicine.

A new dawn for clinical academia?

Teaching

The introduction to this chapter referred to teaching as one of the three core areas of clinical academia, although it has long been the 'Cinderella' of the trio. The Walport report proposes a structured career path for clinical educationalists and recognises that their work is undervalued in medical academia. The report also recommends that further efforts be made for the revision of academic career progression or promotion criteria for such academics, to allow clinical teachers parity with their counterparts in research.[17] This is already happening in progressive medical schools such as Nottingham, Cardiff and St George's, University of London.[26] At last, teaching, which has long been a pivotal role of clinical academics, is being recognised and valued as an important part of an academic's job.

Mentoring

The importance of mentoring in academic medicine has been recognised in the Walport report[17] by senior academics,[8] deaneries[27] and by leading institutions such as the BMA[11] and the Academy of Medical Sciences.[16,28] It has been suggested that gender disparities in promotion may be because women have fewer mentors and professional networks while in the academic medical system.[10] A key function in new and established academic careers is the provision of support for career decisions and advice about publications. There are some exemplary schemes such as that at Imperial College London[7] as well as training programmes for prospective mentors which prepare senior staff for this important role.[27,28]

Currently, mentoring seems to be targeted towards relatively senior staff, although junior staff and medical students would also benefit from contact with an experienced and interested mentor. The scarcity of senior academics to fulfil the role of mentor makes this an ambitious goal.

Role models

Closely associated with the process of mentoring are role models: women and men who have maintained a balance in their work and personal lives, are successful in their careers and who represent a range of routes to 'success' which are not all conventional. Positive role models have been recognised as crucial to encouraging women into academic medicine and into specialties that have traditionally been male-dominated:[8,10,11]

> The problem of recruitment to academic medicine seems likely to become more acute unless women's needs can be accommodated in more flexible career pathways. Attention also needs to be paid to the particular importance of mentors and role models for women in academic medicine.[8]

In 2005 the MASC invited UK academics at all levels to put forward names of role models in academic medicine. The BMA role models report was launched in December 2005.[29] Helen Richardson, a consultant ear, nose and throat surgeon working less than full-time in the north of England writes:

If females continue to reject surgery as a career choice, we will be forced to fill our posts from a (small) pool of men, who may not have the skills or aptitude to make good surgeons. One factor which I think (and have shown through published research) is very important in this discussion is role models – the lack of female surgical role models may result in fewer women going into surgery, which becomes a self perpetuating argument.[4]

The new contract

In 2004 the BMA, through the MASC, successfully negotiated 'a new and unique contract for medical academic staff which binds the Universities and the NHS together in creating, with the academic, an integrated job plan':[15]

This contract is now being used by progressive medical schools to enhance and protect academic staff from overwork and it is a mechanism for positive change. This contract will also enhance co-operation between the NHS and the University sector by offering a 15% pay rise and parity with NHS colleagues.[15]

Improving working lives

At the same time, changing employment practices within the NHS offer a clear direction for clinical academia. These initiatives include self-rostering shifts, annualised-hours agreements, reduced-hours options of different kinds, career breaks and flexible retirement. Annualised hours, in particular, is a simple way of organising the clinical academic job plan, and is supported by the BMA. The 'Improving Working Lives' initiative[30] has also introduced practical help with childcare and other caring responsibilities. We believe that there should be childcare provision available in university and NHS settings for medical academic staff.

The changing workforce

Finally, there has been much coverage in the media of the 'feminisation of medicine'[4,8,31] and its impact. Currently, 61% of medical graduates are women[12] and there is an increasingly female intake into dental schools.[5]

So, could the future of clinical academia be female? At present most female academics remain in positions of little power. In medicine, across the clinical academic grades only 20% of academics are female; at professorial level this drops to 12%, compared to 33% of clinical lecturers.[5] In UK dental schools only 11% of professors are female compared to 45% of clinical lecturers.[5] There are notable exceptions: the presidents of the royal colleges of medicine, radiology and psychiatry are female and the Principal of Warwick Medical School is a woman.

Perhaps a better question, and one that would improve the lot of men and women in clinical academia as well as the populations they serve, be they patients or students, is whether academic medicine and its major partners will seize the opportunities for change offered by the Walport report[17] and the other proposals discussed in this chapter, 'Full implementation of the Walport recommendations will be a major boost to academic medicine and dentistry.'[5] Clinical academia can and should put its own house in order:

> It is clear that the crisis in academic medicine is actually largely caused by factors within academia itself. In challenges such as fair treatment, access and diversity and careers, the medical academic establishment has much to do.[15]

Acknowledgements

Dr Anita Holdcroft, Professor David Oliveira, Professor Martin Roland, Mr Mark Redhead, Ms Deborah Bowman and Dr Liz Arbiter.

Further information

The government has set up a resource centre for women in science, engineering and technology. The website has links to mentoring, role models and advice on returning to work in science, engineering and technology. The Athena project aims to advance women in science, engineering and technology in higher education institutes.

- www.setwomenresource.org.uk
- www.athenaproject.org.uk

References

1 The Medical Women's Federation (2005) (www.medicalwomensfederation.org.uk/eoc_ptw_mwf.htm) (Accessed 16 November 2005)

2 CMAJ (2004) Academic medicine; resuscitation in progress. *CMAJ*. **170**: 309.

3 Sewankando N (2004) Academic medicine and global health responsibilities. *BMJ*. **329**: 752–753.

4 Roberts JH (2005) The feminisation of medicine. *BMJ Careers*. **330**: 13–15.

5 Council of Heads of Medical Schools and Council of Heads and Deans of Dental Schools (2005) *Clinical Academic Staffing Levels in UK Medical and Dental Schools: data update 2004. A Survey by the Council of Heads of Medical Schools and Council of Heads and Deans of Dental Schools. Council of Heads of Medical Schools and Council of Heads and Deans of Dental Schools, England.*

6   Rees M (2005) Speech from the Chairman of the BMA Medical Academic Staff Committee to the Annual Representatives Meeting (ARM), Manchester, June 2005. (www.bma.org.uk/ap.nsf/Content/ARM05chMASC) (Accessed 16 November 2005)

7   British Medical Association (2003) *Encouraging Women to Work in Academic Medicine*. BMA, London.

8   Allen I (2005) Women doctors and their careers: what now? *BMJ*. **331**: 569–572.

9   British Medical Association (2005) *Cohort Study of 1995 Medical Graduates. Tenth Report*. BMA, London.

10 Reichenbach I, Brown H (2004) Gender and academic medicine: impacts on the health workforce. *BMJ*. **329**: 792–795.

11 British Medical Association (2004) *Women in Academic Medicine: Challenges and Issues. A Report by Health Policy and Economic Research Unit*. BMA, London.

12 Research Assessment Exercise 2008: equality briefing for panel chairs, members and secretaries. (www.rae.ac.uk/pubs/2005/02) (Accessed 16 November 2005)

13 Stebbing J, Mandalia S, Portsmouth S *et al.* (2004) A questionnaire survey of stress and bullying in doctors undertaking research. *Postgraduate Medical Journal*. **80**: 93–96.

14 Paice E, Rutter H, Wetherell M *et al.* (2002) Stressful incidents, stress and coping strategies in the pre-registration house officer. *Medical Education*. **36**: 56–65.

15 Rees M (2004) Speech from the Chairman of the BMA Medical Academic Staff Committee to the Annual Representatives Meeting (ARM), Llandudno, June 2004. (www.bma.org.uk/ap.nsf/Content/ARM04chMASC) (Accessed 16 November 2005)

16 Fitzgerald R (2002) National clinician scientist posts. *BMJ Career Focus*. **325**: S101.

17 Academic Careers Sub-Committee of Modernising Medical Careers and the UK Clinical Research Collaboration (2005) *Medically and Dentally Qualified Academic Staff: recommendations for training the researchers and educators of the future*. Academic Careers Sub-Committee of Modernising Medical Careers and the UK Clinical Research Collaboration, England. (www.mmc.nhs.uk/pages/academic) (Accessed 16 November 2005)

18 www.dh.gov.uk (Accessed 16 November 2005)

19 www.wellcome.ac.uk (Accessed 16 November 2005)

20 www.mrc.ac.uk (Accessed 16 November 2005)

21 Bewley S, Davies M, Braude P (2005) Which career first? *BMJ*. **331**: 558–559.

22 Research Assessment Exercise 2008 Consultation on assessment panels' draft criteria and working methods. (www.rae.ac.uk/pubs/2005/04) (Accessed 16 November 2005)

23 www.bma.org.uk/ap.nsf/Content/asessexercise2008

24 Association of University Teachers (2004) *UK Academic Staff 2002–3: gender and research activity in 2001*. RAE, London.

25 Research Assessment Exercise 2008 guidance on submissions Ref RAE 03/2005 (www.rae.ac.uk/pubs/2005/03/) (Accessed 16 November 2005)

26 Kroll L (2005) A flexible job in academic medicine: the Chadburn lectureship. *BMJ Careers*. **331**: 28–29.

27 Doherty C, Hanmer O (2005) Mentoring for doctors in primary and secondary care. In: Hastie A, Hastie N, Jackson N (eds), *Postgraduate Medical Education and Training: a guide for primary and secondary care*. Radcliffe Medical Press, Oxford.

28 Academy of Medical Sciences, mentoring scheme organiser (www.academicmedicine.ac.uk, email: apollo@acmedsci.ac.uk) (Accessed 16 November 2005)

29 BMA (2005) *Role models in academic medicine*. A report by the Health Policy and Economic Research Unit. BMA, London. www.bma.org.uk/masc

30 www.dh.gov.uk/PolicyAndGuidance/HumanResourcesAndTraining/ModelEmployer/ ImprovingWorkingLives/IWLPublications/fs/en?CONTENT_ID=4053583&chk= m%2BN26a (Accessed 16 November 2005)

31 Gray S, Finlay I, Black C (2005) Women doctors and their careers: what now? The changing UK medical workforce's effect on planning and delivery of services. *BMJ*. **331**: 696.

CHAPTER 13

Teaching and training

Induja Bandara, Ann Griffin and Ian Hastie

Why teach?

> No bubble is so iridescent or floats longer than that blown by the successful teacher. (Sir William Osler)

Doctor means 'teacher' in Latin, and teaching is an intrinsic part of the role of the doctor or dentist. We will all be invited to teach at some time in our professional lives, either formally or informally, and your audience could be as diverse as any member of the multi-disciplinary team to any combination of the lay public. The skills of a teacher are of generic use, and though this chapter will be discussing them in a professional capacity, once acquired they will be useful in all your roles. So important is it to our practice that the General Medical Council (GMC) has made it one of the basic tenants of 'Duties of a Doctor', featuring as one of the seven themes of appraisal.[1]

> All doctors have a professional obligation to contribute to the education and training of other doctors, medical students and non-medical healthcare professionals on the team.[2]

To this effect there is a growing ethos to develop the skills of an effective teacher. Teaching allows variety in our daily practice, it stimulates us to keep up to date and we learn from our students, it addresses isolation, is personally rewarding and gives us enthusiasm for our jobs.

What opportunities are there?

There are many and increasing opportunities to teach. Teaching is especially suitable for those who wish to train or work flexibly as it can be easily combined in a planned manner or ad hoc to existing commitments.

Undergraduate teaching

The undergraduate curriculum has changed and continues to change as medicine changes. It is recognised that an undergraduate cannot experience all aspects of medicine and yet, at the same time, needs to gain experience in generic skills such as communication and dealing with patients from different backgrounds. There is now the opportunity to undertake special study modules where a topic is looked at in greater depth. These modules need tutors and are ideal for doctors who are working flexibly. There has been a move away from the teaching being delivered in the teaching hospital to a significant amount now being undertaken in general hospitals and the community. New trends in teaching have been welcomed; in particular, the use of small group teaching in protected time, and this is seen as one of the major strengths of teaching in primary care.

Since the publication of *Tomorrow's Doctors*[3] in 1993, then revised in 2003, community-based teaching has taken a firm foothold in undergraduate medical education, and it now occupies a significant part of the undergraduate curriculum. This has brought in a whole new group of teachers who work in the community and primary care. All aspects of the undergraduate curriculum are represented from a community perspective. This is important, as about 50% of medical students will go on to become primary healthcare physicians and their training should reflect these needs. Almost all specialties are taught with a community focus, and so, as a teacher, you will usually have the ability to pick a topic that suits you. Your experience of problem solving for clinical complaints and knowledge of the common and important topics in community medicine will form the core of your teaching. You are not expected to have expert knowledge. You will also be in a unique environment to support the attitudinal development of younger colleagues at a crucial time. Many new recruits to primary care come from a positive experience of community-based teaching in their undergraduate years. In addition to all this you will be paid to teach at a sessional rate. All medical schools and departments of general practice and primary care will have undergraduate teaching co-ordinators and these are the people to approach for further information. All GPs can apply to teach undergraduate medical students but those in freelance positions will find it difficult without a regular host practice. However, there are often opportunities to teach within the medical school itself or at other sites so it is still worth exploring.

Postgraduate teaching

Foundation programme teaching

As part of *Modernising Medical Careers* (MMC),[4] from August 2005 all newly qualified doctors entered a structured two-year programme, the aims of which

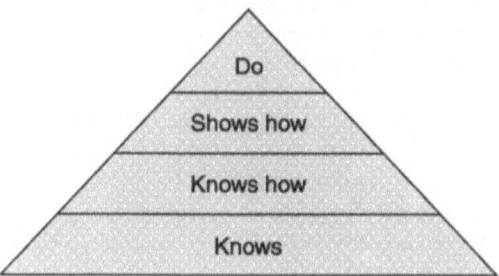

Figure 13.1 Miller's Pyramid.

are to help encourage clinical development, provide additional support and career advice at an early stage for those who need it, facilitate the acquisition of core competencies and translate this to performance, allowing all doctors to develop an overall understanding of the health service, including both primary and secondary care and the interface between them.

Each placement provides trainees with an educational supervisor. For a group of between 20 and 40 foundation trainees there will be a training programme director who will oversee their training, competencies and assessments. There will also be a senior person available to provide career advice and support. All of these posts have part-time commitments so would be suitable for a senior doctor who works flexibly.

A major new theme in education is that of competency-based outcomes: the *doing* rather than *knowing how*, as illustrated by Miller's Pyramid (Figure 13.1).[5]

From this come four new forms of competency-based assessments that teachers will need to be familiar with, and be trained in applying, as they will be an integral part of the foundation programme. The assessment programme (*see* Table 13.1) is intended to be work-based, encouraging formative assessment and professional development as well as documenting the evolution and application of clinical skills.

The first year of the foundation programme (F1) will supplant the present pre-registration house officer (PRHO) training. In the main it will still be based within secondary care, but will entail shorter periods in any one specialty, for example three- or four-month posts. Registration with the GMC will still occur at the end of this year. The second year (F2) will replace the present first year of senior house officer (SHO) training. Competencies that need to be acquired are laid down in the curriculum[4] but the year will take on a different form with at least three different specialties required to be experienced. As well as the traditional acute posts, such as accident and emergency, there are three new areas. There will be opportunities to gain experience in academic medicine, general practice and specialties that have traditionally shown difficulties in recruitment for a variety of reasons: intensive care, histopathology, psychiatry, radiology, microbiology

Table 13.1 Assessment tools for foundation programmes[6]

Type of assessment	Acronym	Tested by	Main focus	Also assesses
Clinical Evaluation Exercise	Mini-CEX	Observing clinical encounters, using a structured checklist	Clinical skills	Professionalism Communication
Direct Observation of Procedural Skills	DOPS	Observing practical procedures using a structured checklist	Practical skills	Professionalism Communication
Peer Assessment Tool and Multiple Source Feedback	Mini-PAT and MSF	Views from a range of clinical colleagues and self-assessment	Professionalism	Clinical care Communication
Case-based Discussion	CBD	Using trainee's entries in patient's notes	Clinical reasoning	Documentation

and virology, public health, allergy, audiology, chemical pathology, clinical genetics, genito-urinary medicine, immunology and nuclear medicine. Each placement will provide the trainee with different experiences so that by the end of the two-year foundation programme each trainee will have acquired the total competencies required.

From August 2006, 55% of the F2 trainees will have experience in general practice, rising to 90% by 2008. This is a major change in that there will now be opportunities for doctors who would not normally be thinking of a career in general practice. This will not only encourage doctors to train in the specialty but also to allow other future specialists to gain from this experience. The main aims of the foundation programme for general practice will be:

- recognition and management of acute illness
- communication skills
- teamwork
- professionalism.

The involvement of general practitioners (GPs) in this programme gives an exciting new and unique opportunity for teaching. F2 doctors can prescribe and will see patients in their own surgeries under supervision. A practice can take on more than one F2 doctor at a time or combine this with undergraduate teaching and/or training a GP registrar. There is no doubt that a positive experience during a F2 GP attachment will encourage those who wish to pursue general practice. Doctors at this key transitional stage in their careers are often looking for role models and mentors to guide the development of their professional practice. Effective educational and personal support can facilitate the development of high calibre physicians aspired to in *Tomorrow's Doctors*.[3]

Established postgraduate teaching

Postgraduate medical education has been subject to change. In general terms we have seen the growing importance put on education through appraisal schemes, the development of the meta-cognitive strategies, self-assessment and reflection as key skills to develop as life-long learners.

Primary care

Working flexibly in general practice can be combined with various types of postgraduate teaching, and practitioners may be asked to assist in the professional development of both clinical and non-clinical members of the primary healthcare team.

Training GP registrars

To become a trainer you will need membership of the Royal College of General Practitioners (RCGP) and in some deaneries a postgraduate certificate in medical education. Regular trainers' workshops and conferences are organised by the deaneries throughout the year for support and development. You need to be established in a regular practice, which needs to be approved according to set criteria in order to take GP registrars.[7] If your registrars are full-time you will need to make arrangements to supervise them adequately in your absence.

Overseas doctors, including refugees

These doctors usually have a wide experience in general practice in their own countries and will need support in acclimatising to our culture and the workings of the National Health Service (NHS). As their supervisor you would help them to identify their specific learning needs, which may be more general, communication-skills orientated and pastoral with an emphasis on facilitating the adaptation to our culture and way of working as opposed to acquiring clinical knowledge.

The clinical experience scheme is a three-month course which aims to enable refugee and overseas doctors to obtain senior house officer (SHO), GP vocational training scheme or GP registrar positions in open competition. It includes a six-week attachment in general practice. Clinical attachments are likely to play an important role in preparing these doctors for employment in the NHS and you may be able to supervise a doctor for a short time in your practice.

Training can be undertaken in general practice while doctors have a limited registration with the GMC. The eligibility criteria for overseas doctors are regularly updated and are available from the national recruitment office for general practice training website.[8] All these GPs may be eligible for higher professional education (HPE) after their training to help their ongoing learning needs and for support (*see* Chapter 6). Guiding and mentoring such doctors may challenge your own perceptions and beliefs.

Secondary care

The organisation of secondary care has undergone major changes and these are continuing. The old structure of single consultant firms working long hours with on-call rotas and learning through apprenticeship has gone. Work now occurs in teams and the European Working Time Directive (EWTD) has reduced the number of maximum working hours for trainees to 56 hours a week, which reduces even further to 48 hours a week in 2009. Many trusts are implementing 'Hospital at Night',[9] where the competencies required at night are assessed and provided by a multi-disciplinary team rather than by several medical on-call teams. MMC has introduced the foundation programme for the first two years, which started in August 2005 and from August 2007 the 'run-through' grade for each specialty comes into being with a more specific training programme taking trainees from the foundation programme through to their certificate of completion of training (CCT).

These changes significantly affect training and learning, and those responsible for promoting learning need a repertoire of new skills and training in how adults learn effectively. The role of simulation in medical training is gathering speed and the airline and nuclear industries have recognised the value of simulation for some time. Medicine has come to this late but now values the great advantages of acquiring skills by simulation before being let loose on patients. In addition to simulators being used before real-life work on patients, simulation has a great role to play in ongoing training, especially working in teams.

In secondary care there have been cohesive organisational efforts to balance service provision and learning. We need to deliver outcome-based training, with appropriate standards and methods of assessment, and have clear educational roles for those supervising training. As an educational or clinical supervisor there is a requirement to assess learning needs, supervise clinical skills, appraise and assess your learners. Supervisors will need to be familiar with effective strategies for work-based learning, giving tutorials, promoting self-direction and reflective practice. All of these are open to the doctor working flexibly.

The Flexible Career Scheme

The Department of Health introduced the Flexible Career Scheme (FCS) in 2002 as part of a wider package of measures to improve doctors' working lives and encourage flexible working within the NHS. The FCS aims to provide additional, funded and supported part-time flexible posts in hospital and general practice, thereby supporting doctors who would otherwise leave the profession because they are unable to find posts that meet their particular working needs.

The hospital scheme has three different opportunities, as follows.

- Doctors in training who wish to take time out of training but maintain their clinical skills by working up to 19 hours per week. This replaces the previous hospital retainer scheme.
- Doctors in career-grade posts, including consultants, who wish to take time out but maintain their clinical skills by working up to 19 hours per week. This also replaces the previous hospital retainer scheme.
- Doctors who wish to return to medicine by working up to 40 hours per week.

Doctors on the hospital FCS will need an educational supervisor or mentor, and a senior doctor who works part-time would be ideal as they would have personal experience of not wanting to work full-time in medicine.

The GP FCS provides the opportunity to work up to five sessions a week in a flexible post and general practice still has a GP Retainer Scheme where GPs can work up to four sessions per week. The GP Returner Scheme is designed to facilitate the return of qualified GPs to the NHS. These GPs may have been out of medical practice altogether or working as doctors in areas other than general practice and inevitably their learning needs will be unique and vary accordingly.

All three GP schemes have prominent educational components and the practice needs to allocate an educational supervisor who will have a mentoring role and be involved in the facilitation of their continuing professional development. The whole practice will be involved in the support of these doctors, as much of the learning will be work-based. These GPs are a diverse group with various types and length of experience and your educational role will vary accordingly. Some will require a period of refresher training of up to six months' full-time, tailormade to training requirements identified for each doctor. These GPs may need help in boosting their confidence, enhancing their problem-solving skills, reforming working networks and working independently. Typical learning needs include clinical placements, information technology and practice management training, consultation and communications skills, time management, assertiveness and negotiation skills, interview skills, practice finance management. Educational supervisors for GP returners will need the same skills as trainers and receive the same support and remuneration. Protected learning time should be made available for the GP educator and learner to meet on a regular basis for tutorials, which should be learner-led, such as discussions about case management, significant events, reflective practice and so on. Other skills, such as mentoring, are invaluable, defined for doctors in training as:

A process whereby an experienced highly regarded, empathic person [the mentor] guides another individual [the mentee] in the development and re-examination of their own ideas, learning and personal and professional development. This is achieved by listening and talking in confidence.[10]

How to become a medical educator

The most effective way of developing your teaching skills is a balance between the theory and practice of learning and teaching. With a planned shortening of time in specialist training grades, and MMC, which aims 'to develop demonstrably competent doctors who are skilled at communicating and working as effective members of a team'[4] there is a move away from the apprenticeship model. Those responsible for promoting learning need a repertoire of new skills and training in how adults learn effectively. There is a growing trend towards professionalism in teaching and with this an increasing availability of teacher training courses. They fall into two main categories.

Introduction to teaching

These courses are usually two or three days in duration and cover basic knowledge on adult learning. They are useful for acquiring practical skills on how to make teaching effective; for example, lesson planning, assessing students and giving feedback. These courses are extremely useful to increase confidence and acquire some of the technical skills to implement when teaching. They are an excellent preparation for beginning to teach in primary and/or secondary care and the postgraduate deaneries and universities run such courses. There may be further training depending on who you plan to teach; for example, in under-graduate education specific training will be needed about the chosen course and its curriculum.

In general practice in order to be an approved educational supervisor you will be required to attend regular meetings throughout the year, in the form of learning sets, so you can develop your teaching skills whilst actively engaged in supporting your learner.

Accredited courses

There are further courses up to diploma or masters degree level, which are accredited through the universities. These are open to all disciplines, including both primary and secondary care doctors. For those wishing to become a GP trainer a postgraduate certificate in education (PGCE) may be needed in some deaneries and there are two main ways of achieving this. GPs can enrol in either taught courses or in distant learning programmes. The advantage with the distance learning packages is that they very much suit a flexible working pattern.

The postgraduate certificate can also be extended to a diploma or masters degree in medical education if the bug really bites hard.

The Higher Education Academy

Membership of the Higher Education Academy[11] is recognition of excellence in teaching and learning. Entry is gained by achieving the postgraduate certificate or via the individual entry route. This allows applicants to submit evidence directly to the Academy, demonstrating that they have satisfied the criteria for registration through professional experience. Once accepted the doctor will be able to use the post-nominal letters ILTM/A

Developing as an educator

Having gained the knowledge, skills and attitudes of an effective teacher by combining the theory and practice of teaching and learning, the next stage is to keep up to date and develop further by becoming a reflective practitioner. The reflective practitioner will use a host of sources to gain feedback on their teaching; good examples include student evaluations, patients' feedback and the use of peers or colleagues. Using these sources helps your own personal reflection on the teaching process and leads to the development of your skills. Good practice includes developing a teaching portfolio in which is included your feedback, self-evaluations and documentation, as evidence of the changes and developments of your teaching.

You may want to develop your skills by taking on other roles which support learning; for example, being an appraiser, mentor or tutor. Once you have developed the skills of an educator, you will be surprised by the range of invitations to teach that are offered to you: invitations from schools, institutions of higher education, groups of other professionals and the lay public. We hope that you will find this additional facet to your work rewarding and satisfying.

When a simple, earnest spirit animates a college, there is no appreciable interval between the teacher and the taught – both are in the same class, the one a little more advanced than the other. (William Osler, 1905)

References

1   General Medical Council (2001) *Good Medical Practice*. GMC, London.

2   General Medical Council (1999) *The Doctor as a Teacher*. GMC, London.

3   General Medical Council (2003) *Tomorrow's Doctors: recommendations on undergraduate medical education*. GMC, London.

4   www.mmc.nhs.uk

5   Miller GE (1990) The assessment of clinical skills/competence/performance. *Academic Medicine.* **65**: 563–567.

6   Davies H, Archer J and Heard S (2005) Assessment tools for foundation programmes – a practical guide. *General Practice BMJ Careers.* **330**: 195–6.

7   Joint Committee on Postgraduate Training for General Practice (2001). *The Selection and Re-selection of GP Trainers.* JCPTGP, London.

8   www.gprecruitment.org.uk

9   www.modern.nhs.uk/workingtime/ 17048/WhatisHospitalatNight/1_1.pdf

10 Standing Committee on Postgraduate Medical and Dental Education (1998) *Supporting Doctors and Dentists at Work: an enquiry into mentoring.* SCOPME, London.

11 www.heacademy.ac.uk

CHAPTER 14

The portfolio general practitioner

Nav Chana and John Spicer

Introduction

The nature of the way in which doctors work in general practice has changed. At a structural level, the medical workforce itself has changed. One in three general practitioners (GPs) is a woman, and two-thirds of medical students wanting to go into general practice are women. Their desire for family-friendly working hours, such as part-time, flexible working, term-time only, are now also being adopted by their male colleagues. Almost one-fifth of all GP principals now work part-time in general practice.[1]

The traditional model of GP 'principals', working full-time in one practice for their working life seems outdated. Part-time clinical responsibilities, with diversification into teaching, research, developing special clinical interests or simply striving to achieve an appropriate work–life balance now seem to be key factors.

In other primary care disciplines, colleagues have become used to informal career pathways demonstrating 'width rather than length'.[2] Despite a formal career structure, the need to accommodate 'portfolio working' in general practice is clear.

What is portfolio working?

The terms 'portfolio working' or 'portfolio doctor' are just a few among a veritable word salad of recently emerged descriptors for new ways of working in general practice. It is suggested that the following definition for portfolio working is adopted: 'A doctor who has more than one source of earned income'.

So what is in discussion is someone who may work across several different fields within or outside medicine. The archetypal GP who cared for patients over many years in the same community as a sole practitioner is at an opposite pole from the portfolio GP.

Handy[3] introduced the notion of portfolio working as an alternative to linear career paths, and as a response to changing social patterns. In fact, general practice has traditionally been characterised by an early plateau effect: the achievement of principal status. Perhaps another driver to a more varied career is represented by diversification after that stage. Harrison[4] sets these general trends in a post-modern context of flexibility and uncertainty applying as much to GPs as anyone else.

Benefits of a portfolio career

A national survey of job satisfaction and retirement intentions among GPs found that the proportion of doctors intending to leave general practice rose from 14% in 1998 to 22% in 2001.[5] It has been suggested that doctors might be encouraged to stay working in the National Health Service (NHS) for longer by offering them more flexible working patterns, reducing their workload with age and offering them greater professional freedom.[6] Portfolio working clearly represents an option for this group of doctors.

Outside medicine, some common themes emerge which characterise and motivate portfolio working. A degree of control over one's workload is common, linked to the ability to control whom one works with. There is variety and unpredictability available, which may help to minimise the 'burn-out' effect. Of course, for some people, these qualities may be interpreted negatively and add to a certain loneliness, uncertainty, insecurity or irritant need to network to find work.

The obituary of Colin McEvedy provides an exemplar. Not only was he a psychiatrist and researcher, but also an original map-maker of the ancient world.[7] Few can achieve such an enormous spread of knowledge and skills.

A more typical pattern of activities would lie more or less within a clinical, educational or managerial sphere.[8] Harris describes an example of the typical working week of a portfolio GP, as listed below:[9]

- running evening sessions for two patient groups
- helping to organise the Bath area obstetrics service
- working as a GP trainer
- teaching medical students
- working as a course organiser (lecturer at University of Bath)
- examining for the MRCGP (four weeks a year)
- representing GP educators in negotiations with the Department of Health
- doing a masters degree (MMEd)
- writing a book.

The positive side of carrying multiple responsibilities is the satisfaction that they bring individually and collectively: the working week is varied and stimulating.

It can change from week to week, and repetition or boredom is rarely an issue.

By definition, GPs are generalists, and therefore moving into roles beyond solely clinical practice is actually a natural and appropriate development. The formal aspects of training to be a GP with special interest (GpwSI) may illustrate a particular clinical interest, perhaps as a hangover from a previous career path or training experience, or a broadening of practice over time. Nonetheless, when the professional base is broad, diversification can be seen as a natural progression.

Problems associated with portfolio working

It is tempting to think in the terms described above that the working week can be neatly divided into sections: a quota of sessions or days for this job, or that job. Certainly, this may happen, but the reality is likely to be different. Thus, by the very nature of holding several responsibilities, more effort, time and sometimes stress is engendered.[10] That precious work–life balance can be threatened. The various jobs are more than the sum of their parts.

Some issues need further consideration. First, even though the working week may be notionally divided, it is easy for issues coming up from one area of responsibility to invade another. A solution, though by no means the only one, is to multi-task. Email is a typical example of this.

Second, there may be transferable skills between the variety of tasks performed: working as a teacher has obvious overlaps with working as a clinician by virtue of communication skills, clinical content and more.

Third, to maintain professional skills in several areas at once is inviting the potential erosion of free time. After all, to retain and develop the knowledge and skills of general practice requires an irreducible commitment of time whether one works part-time or not. Applying that principle to the list of GP activities above will generate an enormous time investment in continuing professional development, review and appraisal. Despite the fact that GPs are known to be effective self-directed learners,[11] that commitment can sometimes be overwhelming across many domains of learning.

Fourth, it has been noted that GPs who run portfolio careers may suffer financially as a result of doing so, and almost always experience conflict with their (GP) partners.[12] This may be a significant disincentive for many GPs, and a formal career structure to try and solve these problems is needed. Young and Leese[13] suggested possible solutions to the retention crisis in general practice. This includes offering a wider choice of long-term career paths, programmes of professional development and training, widening the scope of remuneration and range of contract conditions, and greater choice and flexibility in working hours.

Portfolio working in the new NHS

The requirement for GPs to work part-time, flexibly and develop portfolio careers inevitably restricts individual patients' access to their personal GP. In addition, this style of working clearly imposes the need to recruit more doctors to deliver the service, but the situation is exacerbated by the current shortages of GPs allowing prospective salaried GPs to negotiate better personal terms. All of this is perhaps good for individual doctors but, in turn, may threaten the strengths of primary care (that is, continuous, comprehensive and fully 'joined up'),[14] and may have an adverse effect on patient satisfaction.

The government's plurality agenda makes it clear that patient choice, competition and contestability are key principles underpinning future service reform.[15] In the new General Medical Services (nGMS) contract there is specific provision for practices to opt out of providing some services. Where this occurs care will need to be provided by other providers.

There is now scope to introduce new NHS organisations, through the Specialist Personal Medical Services (SPMS) contractual arrangements,[16] and private companies, through the Alternative Provider Medical Services (APMS) contractual arrangements.[17] New contractual arrangements for the wider primary care professionals, such as pharmacists, present another vehicle for change. Furthermore, secondary care providers, for example foundation trusts, may well seek to extend their provision of services into areas traditionally delivered in primary care to secure activity and therefore income.

If the new providers prove as least as effective as existing primary care services but more willing to reform and embrace the changes demanded by government and patients, it may not be long until they encroach into core general practice services. Given the high unit cost of GPs, the increasingly contractual nature of the way GPs work and the difficulty in recruiting more GPs to provide the same service, commissioners of primary care may well ask the reasonable question: Does the service need more GPs?

Portfolio working and generalism

The recent Department of Health paper, *Commissioning a Patient-led NHS*,[18] underlines the importance of practice-based commissioning in redesigning services which are configured along patient care pathways. The emphasis will be on developing an effective skill mix of health professionals focused on the needs of the patients. Attention will focus on patients with complex needs, who are at high risk of hospitalisation, to create more planned and proactive care delivered in the community. New species of health professionals, such as community matrons, are being developed to take on the case management of these patients.

It is known that increasing the number of generalist physicians reduces hospital utilisation.[13] An appropriately trained GP brings to the table key skills that are crucial in managing this group of patients: the ability to discriminate undifferentiated symptoms against a background of knowledge of the patient (therefore to manage uncertainty and risk) and the ability to manage patients with complex problems and co-morbidities. The new RCGP curriculum[19] outlines these requirements in defining the core competences of being a GP. However, it is arguable that the more diverse the activities of a portfolio GP (including GP specialisation), the greater the risk of losing precisely those skills that define the unique additional contribution a GP can make to the future enhanced primary care team.

Conclusion

Portfolio working has undoubted benefits to the individual, and benefits the NHS in its current forms by offering a strategy for retaining the existing GP workforce. However, in light of changes to the structure and function of the new NHS, it is important to consider the potential implications of adopting the portfolio approach more widely.

Patients need support in the health and life decisions that they have to take, and the vast majority of them currently still like it to come from their 'own' doctor.[20] It is important therefore that GPs, in defining the way they wish to work, do not swing the pendulum so far that patients are forced to seek alternative providers of primary healthcare.

References

1   Department of Health (2002) *General Practitioner Recruitment, Retention and Vacancy Survey 2002 England and Wales*. London: Government Statistical Service.

2   Murray E and Simpson J (eds) (2000) *Professional Development and Management for Therapists: an introduction*. Blackwell Science, Oxford.

3   Handy C (1995) *The Age of Unreason*. Random House, London.

4   Harrison J (1998) Post modern influences. In: Harrison J and Van Zwanenberg T (eds), *GP Tomorrow*. Radcliffe Medical Press, Oxford.

5   Sibbald B, Bojke C and Gravelle H (2003) National survey of job satisfaction and retirement intentions among general practitioners in England. *BMJ*. **326**: 22–24.

6   Davidson J, Lambert T, Parkhouse J, Evans J and Goldacre M (2001) Retirement intentions of doctors who qualified in the United Kingdom in 1974: postal questionnaire survey. *Journal of Public Health Medicine*. **23**: 323–328.

7   Obituary. (2005) *Independent*, 30 August.

8   Thornett A, Chambers R and Baker M (2003) Pick 'n' mix career options for GPs. *BMJ Careeer Focus*. **326**: 213–215.

9   www.mharris.eurobell.co.uk/resource/lovegp/portfolio.htm

10 Houghton A (2005) Stress and time management for people with multiple responsibilities. *BMJ Career Focus*. **331**: 30.

11 Bandara I and Calvert G (2002) General practitioners: uncelebrated adult learners – a qualitative study. *Education for Primary Care*. **13**: 370–378.

12 Archard G (2003) *A GP Workforce for All the Talents: a discussion document on a possible career structure for portfolio general practice*. NHS Alliance, London.

13 Young R and Leese B (1999) Recruitment and retention of general practitioners in the UK: what are the problems and solutions? *Br J Gen Pract*. **49**: 829–333.

14 Starfield B (1998) *Primary Care: balancing health needs, services, and technology*. Oxford University Press, New York.

15 Department of Health (2003) *Building on the Best: choice, responsiveness and equity in the NHS*. HMSO, London.

16 Department of Health (2003) *Sustaining Innovation Through New PMS Arrangements*. HMSO, London.

17 Department of Health (2004) *Alternative Provider Medical Services (APMS) Guidance*. HMSO, London.

18 Department of Health (2005) *Commissioning a Patient-led NHS*. Department of Health, London. (Available at www.doh.gov.uk)

19 Royal College of General Practitioners (2006) The Core Statement – *Being a General Practitioner*. RCGP, London.

20 MORI (2003) *Exploring Patient Choice*. MORI. www.mori.com/polls/2003/bupa.shtml

CHAPTER 15

Sabbaticals

Anne Hastie

Introduction

Working as a doctor or dentist in the National Health Service (NHS) is demanding, and once an individual is appointed to a consultant or practitioner post they may stay in the same job for 20 or more years. In these circumstances a lack of stimulation may lead to demoralisation, and a sabbatical allows a period of recreation or the opportunity to develop new professional skills. Younger doctors and dentists may wish to take time out between jobs to pursue other interests, travel or work abroad. General practice registrars who constructed a three-month sabbatical to undertake an educational activity of their own choice viewed the experience positively, with both the practice doctors and patients noticing a positive change in the registrars when they returned to work.[1]

Research in other professional areas suggests that sabbaticals confer considerable benefits, in particular in relation to reducing stress and avoiding burn-out. Jarecky and Sandifer found that 80% of a medical school faculty who undertook a sabbatical viewed their experience favourably and the benefits in terms of research and publication were substantial.[2] Tait,[3] and Evans *et al.*[4] suggested the importance of study leave in addressing the problem of burn-out. Feldman, in the USA, demonstrates that undertaking a sabbatical not only enables physicians to learn new skills, but also provides relief from burn-out and valuable time for introspection.[5] Lack of study leave has been found to be related to greater disillusionment with general practice, and Braithwaite and Ross suggest that opportunities for continuing education could play an important role in alleviating this.[6]

Research in the area of recruitment and retention within general practice identified high levels of dissatisfaction associated with rising levels of stress relating to the 1990 NHS contract changes, and increasing disillusionment with the role of the general practitioner (GP).[7,8] Kmietowicz[9] found that a quarter of UK GPs wanted to leave the profession and many more were planning to take early retirement. As O'Dowd[10] pointed out, doctors suffering from burn-out often feel they have nowhere to go because opportunities for mid-career development are not integral to the GP career structure. The intention of some GPs to retire early is linked to job dissatisfaction, and Sibbald has suggested that if job satisfaction can be increased more GPs will be retained.[11] Young and Leese have identified the importance to retention by enabling GPs to develop their career paths.[12]

Organising a sabbatical takes time and motivation, with many obstacles to overcome, but the benefits can be considerable to individuals, their families, colleagues and patients. There are several ways in which a sabbatical can be taken, including:

- unpaid leave
- paid leave
- prolonged study leave for GPs
- gaps between jobs
- out of programme experience.

All NHS doctors and dentists need to be aware that taking more than three months' unpaid leave could mean a break in service and may result in a reduction in benefits such as maternity or sick pay. Service or training of up to 12 months overseas may not count as a break in service and doctors and dentists should investigate their individual situation before making their plans.

Voluntary work

There are opportunities to do voluntary medical work in the UK and abroad. Organisations such as the Red Cross, Oxfam and other relief agencies value the help of British doctors and dentists, particularly those with skills in specialties where the need is great, such as anaesthetics and surgical procedures. Many GPs and hospital doctors have experience in medical education, which is in demand from countries that are trying to improve their service provision through education and training. Medical royal colleges and postgraduate deaneries are often asked to help find doctors to give advice and expertise with new projects.

Funding

The ideal is to be able to take paid leave. If this is not possible then travel grants, scholarships, sponsorship and other awards may be available for doctors and dentists planning a sabbatical. The British Medical Association (BMA), the World Health Organization (WHO) and medical royal colleges offer various awards. Research grants may be available from within the NHS, pharmaceutical industry or independent bodies such as the King's Fund. Prolonged study leave is available for GPs and is discussed in more detail later in this chapter, although the funding is cash-limited.

Hospital doctors and dentists

There is no specific provision for consultants and senior career grade staff to be granted sabbatical leave, although employers have the discretion to grant paid or unpaid leave. Employers are also able to grant special leave to undertake a period of study leave abroad. A more formalised access to sabbaticals has been suggested but has yet to be successfully negotiated. Junior hospital doctors and dentists may decide to take time out between jobs to take a sabbatical, which might include travel abroad.

Out of programme experience

An out of programme experience (OOPE) is currently (2006) available to specialist registrars and allows time out of a clinical training programme whilst retaining a training number. It has not yet been agreed at what stage in the training an OOPE can be taken when the new run-through training begins in 2007. Trainees are required to obtain formal approval from their postgraduate dean, who will require the agreement of their educational supervisor, training programme director with responsibility for their specialty and chair of the specialty training committee (STA). The maximum time allowed out of programme is normally three years and trainees should explore with the appropriate royal college or faculty whether any or all of their requested time out can count towards their certificate of completion of training (CCT). Extensions beyond three years will only be allowed in exceptional circumstances and will need further written approval from the postgraduate dean.

Requests for OOPEs are usually for research, clinical experience in a different setting (including abroad) or for personal reasons. Trainees should normally make requests at least six months prior to starting their OOPE and a minimum of three months is required in order to give notice to their employer. Trainees need to give at least six months' notice of their intention to return to their training programme and they should liaise with their training programme director to organise their re-entry into clinical training. If the OOPE is in research or a clinical placement trainees will need to return a record of in-service training assessment (RITA) form F at the end of each year that they are out of programme. This will need to be accompanied by a report of the progress in the research or clinical placement.

Trainees should look at their postgraduate deanery website for further information and application forms. Some deaneries, including London, will allow an OOPE of up to one year for doctors on their GP vocational training schemes. GP trainees should explore whether any or all of their requested time out can count towards their training and if it is then a letter of confirmation is required as part of the OOPE documentation.

NHS practitioners

Doctors and dentists working as practitioners in primary care are either self-employed or salaried. Some enlightened partnerships have an agreement in their partnership contract that partners can take a sabbatical to do anything they choose while continuing to draw their partnership profit. The length and frequency varies according to individual partnership agreements and ranges from one to 12 months every five to 10 years. A savings account can be set up with monthly deposits to build up sufficient funds to support sabbaticals. In other practices the partner taking a sabbatical will be responsible for finding and funding a locum. Practice exchanges used to be popular but legislation now requires all GPs working in the UK to hold the appropriate certification so this has become a difficult way to organise a sabbatical.

Early planning is essential and GPs will need to get permission from the primary care trust (PCT), which will want to ensure that patient services continue to be fully provided, which may mean employing a locum. Those doctors and dentists who are salaried will need to obtain permission from their employing practice to take a sabbatical and if granted may have to take unpaid leave.

Prolonged study leave for GPs

This is probably the most generous way of taking a sabbatical in the NHS and is unique to general practice. Prolonged study leave provides GPs with the opportunity to develop knowledge and skills in an area of personal career interest. This could include studying for a higher degree, enhancing their role through the development of specialist medical knowledge, teaching or academic research. Prolonged study leave cannot be used to take college exams such as the MRCGP as the NHS does not directly fund membership of professional organisations. However, there is nothing to prevent GPs using prolonged study leave to prepare themselves and their practices for becoming a trainer or using information from their prolonged study leave research to support an application for MRCGP or FRCGP.

Although comparatively few GPs apply for prolonged study leave there is significant expenditure involved for the PCT if it funds the educational and locum allowances for the absent GP. Prolonged study leave can be taken on a full- or part-time basis, although part-time GPs would only be able to apply for prolonged study leave for the sessions they would normally work in the practice:

- minimum 10 weeks or 50 days (pro rata for part-time GPs)
- maximum 12 months or 260 days (pro rata for part-time GPs).

GPs who undertake prolonged study leave may face the accusation that they have 'retreated from the harsh reality of general practice',[13] and prolonged study leave is seen by many as an option taken by GPs who want to leave, rather than remain in, general practice. However, recent research has demonstrated the effectiveness of prolonged study leave in refreshing and renewing the interest and commitment of GPs to general practice.[14,15] On returning to practice, many GPs developed their roles by taking on additional appointments such as committee membership or advisory posts enabling them to enhance their careers and benefit their local healthcare community.

The greatest benefit reported by GPs who have done prolonged study leave is a sense of personal satisfaction and development with a broader perspective of their career and a renewed enthusiasm for primary care. Many GPs report increased confidence in their skills and abilities resulting in the provision of better services for patients. If government changes have had the effect of threatening the traditional values and job satisfaction associated with general practice, prolonged study leave may help to redress this by offering GPs the opportunity to regain a sense of autonomy in the development of their careers and a renewed interest in their work. Training for general practice currently provides little experience in research or business management.[16] As a greater emphasis is placed on evidence-based medicine, and management skills become increasingly important, the opportunity to undertake prolonged study leave provides a valuable opportunity for GPs to develop these skills.

Funding for prolonged study leave

Until April 2004, prolonged study leave was funded by the Department of Health from a central non-cash-limited budget but was only available to GP principals. Providing the application for prolonged study leave gained approval, the GP principal would automatically receive the funding, but with an increasing number of GPs working freelance and in salaried posts this became unfair. The new general medical services contract (nGMS) introduced on 1 April 2004 allows all GPs to be able to apply for prolonged study leave funding. However, the budget has now been devolved to PCTs as part of their total budget allocation and is cash-limited.

Under paragraph 15.1 of the Statement of Financial Entitlements (SFE) doctors who are performers of primary medical services under a General Medical Services (GMS) contract may be entitled to take prolonged study leave, and in these circumstances the contractor for whom they have been providing primary medical services may be entitled to two payments:

- an educational allowance, to be forwarded to the doctor taking prolonged study leave
- the cost of, or a contribution towards the cost of, a locum or deputy.

A locum must be employed and the locum allowance cannot just be added to the partnership profits. The locum allowance is paid on a pro rata basis for part-time study; for example, if a GP is on prolonged study leave for four sessions per week the PCT will probably pay 4/9ths of the maximum of the locum allowance. The education allowance will be paid in full for up to 12 months, including part-time study as this allowance is a contribution towards the extra cost of study (i.e. course fees, books and travel expenses). However, the PCT has to determine that prolonged study leave payments are affordable with regard to the PCT's annual budgetary targets, which means that the PCT can refuse funding on the grounds of affordability. Doctors providing Personal Medical Services (PMS) should also be able to apply to their PCT for prolonged study leave funding, subject to the same constraints.

If another organisation contributes towards the cost of a GP's prolonged study leave it is likely to affect the allowances paid by the PCT through abatement. If any payments or grants are received after the prolonged study leave application has been accepted it is essential that GPs discuss this with the PCT. Failure to do this may result in the repayment of all allowances paid or be viewed as fraudulent.

Making an application

GPs considering applying for prolonged study leave should first obtain information from the website of their postgraduate medical deanery. If the GP wants to proceed with an application it would then be sensible to approach their PCT to see if it would be willing to fund the period of proposed prolonged study leave providing an application was approved by the postgraduate deanery. The GP should seek the advice of the Director of Postgraduate General Practice (DPGPE) or nominated deputy who should be able to give valuable guidance. Retrospective applications are not considered.

The following paperwork needs to be completed in full:

- application form
- declaration from the practice
- declaration from the PCT
- letter of support from the educational institution or supervisor.

In addition, applicants should write an executive summary of their proposed prolonged study leave, which should include details of:

- benefits to themselves
- benefits to their practice
- benefits to their locality
- benefits to the NHS as a whole.

The application form and supporting documents should be sent to the local DPGPE for approval. There is a national prolonged study leave panel consisting of four experienced UK DPGPEs who will assess difficult or complex applications at the request of the local DPGPE and this takes at least six weeks. If a GP is successful in gaining educational approval for prolonged study leave the GP and PCT will be informed. At the end of a period of prolonged study leave the GP must write a report of 3000–5000 words summarising their achievements during prolonged study leave and send it to the DPGPE and PCT. This ensures that public money has been used effectively.

Summary

A sabbatical can refresh and retain doctors and dentists, but opportunities are variable. GPs have the best opportunity through prolonged study leave but it is dependent on their PCT having available funding. Paid leave for a sabbatical can be cost effective if the doctor or dentist might otherwise leave the profession through burn-out. Sabbaticals that enhance the professional skills of doctors or dentists will benefit their organisation and patients.

References

1   Gibbs T and Harvey J (1999) Sabbaticals for general practitioners: will they solve an educational problem? *Education for General Practice*. **10**: 449–455.

2   Jarecky RK and Sandifer MG (1986) Faculty members' evaluations of sabbaticals. *Journal of Medical Education*. **61**: 803–807.

3   Tait I (1987) Take a sabbatical from general practice. *BMJ*. **295**: 644–646.

4   Evans A, Ford J and Bahrami J (2002) Prolonged study leave: who takes it, and what is it for? *Education for Primary Care*. **13**: 451–456.

5   Feldman MK (1999) Physician sabbaticals can provide relief from burnout, a chance to learn new skills and time for introspection. *Minnesota Medicine*. **82**: 23–24.

6   Braithwaite A and Ross A (1988) Satisfaction and job stress in general practice. *Family Practice*. **5**: 83–93.

7   Appleton K, House A and Dowell A (1998) A survey of job satisfaction, sources of stress and psychological symptoms among general practitioners in Leeds. *Br J Gen Pract*. **48**: 1959–1563.

8   Myerson S (1993) The effects of policy change on family doctors: stress in general practice under the new contract. *Journal of Management in Medicine*. **7**: 7–25.

9   Kmietowicz Z (2001) Quarter of GPs want to quit, BMA survey shows. *BMJ*. **323**: 887–888.

10   O'Dowd T (1987) To burn or rust out in general practice. *Journal of the Royal College of General Practitioners*. **37**: 290–291.

11   Sibbald B, Bojke C and Gravelle H (2003) National survey of job satisfaction and retirement intentions among general practitioners in England. *BMJ*. **326**: 22–24.

12 Young R and Leese B (1999) Recruitment and retention of general practitioners in the UK: what are the problems and solutions? *Br J Gen Pract.* **49**: 829–833.

13 Handysides S (1994) Enriching careers in general practice: is change the problem or the solution. *BMJ.* **308**: 32–34.

14 Hastie A and Clark R (2004) An assessment of prolonged study leave. *Education for Primary Care.* **15**: 378–382.

15 Hutchins A, Hastie A, Starkey C *et al.* (2005) An investigation into the benefits of prolonged study leave undertaken by general practitioners. *Education for Primary Care.* **16**: 57–65.

16 Handysides S (1994) Enriching careers in general practice: building morale through personal development. *BMJ.* **308**: 114–116.

CHAPTER 16

Leadership, management and the flexible career

Tim Swanwick

Introduction

What role do doctors have in the management and leadership of the National Health Service (NHS)? Should physicians confine themselves to clinical activity? Should individual patient outcomes be our only concern, or do we have a role in managing the system, in enhancing and redesigning services and improving the patient experience? Where are the clinical leaders of the future; in the consulting room and clinic, or in the back offices and administration blocks of our practices and hospitals? This chapter explores the nature of management and leadership, and argues that in a perpetually modernising NHS, the need for clinicians' involvement in these distinct, but inter-related, activities has never been greater. In particular, the focus is on the roles and professional responsibilities of doctors working flexibly. Despite their distinctive characteristics – always part-time, often female – it is hoped to demonstrate the importance of clinicians' involvement in service development, that management is an activity not a profession and that leadership is everyone's responsibility.

Setting the scene: the NHS today

'Change is the only constant.' The words of the Greek philosopher Heraclitus are as relevant today as they were in 500 BC. In fact, in the NHS the pace of change, far from being constant, is accelerating, as one of the world's largest organisations struggles to adapt to new technologies, increased patient expectations and the prevailing political dogmas of consumer choice and contestability.

The current wave of change, at least in England, originates in the Department of Health publication, *The NHS Plan*,[1] which articulated a 10-year vision for the NHS; an NHS fit for purpose, designed around the needs of patients. *The NHS Plan*[1] outlined how increased funding and reform would redress geographical inequalities, improve service standards and extend patient choice. This would be achieved through 'a new delivery system for the NHS' with a greater emphasis on primary care (one-stop health centres, public–private finance deals for new premises, development of practitioners with special interests) and changes for social services and NHS staff groups. *Shifting the Balance of Power*[2] set out a programme of change to enable implementation of *The NHS Plan*, notably through the creation of primary care trusts (PCTs), to whom was given responsibility to commisison healthcare, provide local services and improve the health of the population. The *NHS Improvement Plan*[3] reaffirmed the vision for high-quality personal services to individual patients and, at the same time, shifted the emphasis from treatment to prevention. Meanwhile, in secondary care the Health and Social Care Act (2003) established NHS foundation trusts: not-for-profit public benefit corporations with local ownership and involvement of patients, the public and staff.

Within the last 18 months, *Commisioning a Patient-led NHS*[4] has described how the roles and configurations of PCTs and strategic health authorities (SHAs) will be redefined, and reinstitutes practice-based commissioning of services – a system dismantled by the same government only eight years previously. Elsewhere in the UK similar shifts in emphasis have occurred, perhaps not with quite the same manic enthusiasm for restucturing, on the back of other country-specific policies: *A Healthier Future: A Twenty Year Vision for Health and Wellbeing in Northern Ireland 2005–2025*,[5] Scotland's *Our National Plan: A Plan for Action, A Plan for Change*[6] and *Improving Health in Wales: A Plan for the NHS in Wales*.[7]

Two major themes run through all these changes: first, recognition that if the NHS is to be truly patient-responsive, radical service redesign is required and, second, that this can only be achieved by bringing clinical leadership and management closer to the patient. Improving the NHS for the better depends on changing systems, not just working harder within them. System improvement requires the involvement of all those working within it and clinicians are ideally placed to lead that process. As far back as 1983, Sir Roy Griffiths, then Managing Director of Sainsbury and adviser to Margaret Thatcher on NHS management, highlighted that 'The nearer that the management process gets to the patient, the more important it becomes for doctors to be looked upon as the natural managers.'[8]

So are doctors the natural managers of the health service? Twenty years on from the Griffiths Report,[8] the discourse has changed and management tends to be viewed as a lowly function, akin to the American concept of adminstration, but the need is still there. Clinicians working at the front line are being invited by the government to lead on service reform through foundation trusts, primary care commissioning groups and new and innovative constellations of providers. Effective service management is required, reframed as a call for clinical leadership, a more sexy term altogether. Indeed, we would probably all prefer to be seen as a leader than a manager but as we shall see, the two concepts are inextricably linked.

'Leadership' and 'management' are highly contested terms that mean different things to diffferent people. So before moving on to discuss just how doctors working flexibly can involve themselves in the redesign of today's NHS, let us consider both concepts in more detail.

What is management?

Management is concerned with 'getting things done through influencing others'.[9] Looking after the complexities of today with a primary concern for the immediate operational environment. Management can be seen to revolve around six core tasks:

- planning
- allocating resources
- co-ordinating the work of others
- motivating staff
- monitoring output
- taking responsibility for the process.

Management, then, is about getting things done and doing things right. Managers focus on the process, not the substance, of issues and in doing so may be seen as inflexible, detached and sometimes manipulative.[10] Management is a transactional process in which those that follow the manager do so in their own self-interest, in return for some reward or punishment, be it financial or related to job prospects or prestige. Effective management is clearly essential for the smooth running of organisations, without it they would degenerate into an anarchic melée of competing self-interest groups. In healthcare, a mounting body of evidence points to the fact that poorly managed organisations fail patients, frustrate staff, deliver poor-quality care and are ill-equipped to adapt to the changing demands of the environment in which they operate.[11]

But management, as defined here, is not enough on its own. The tasks described in the list above assume a degree of core stability and that the organisation's strategic direction is clear and unambiguous. But, as we have seen, the NHS is a complex, ever-shifting organisation in which neither of these two assumptions hold true. Making sense of the world, setting direction and taking others with you in an environment of constant change requires something more, and it is to this missing ingredient: leadership, that we will turn to next.

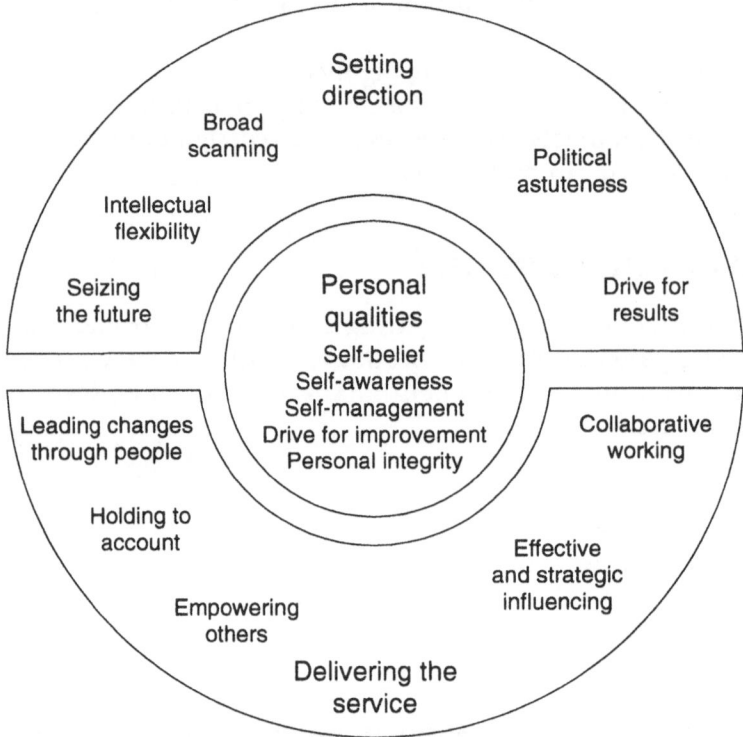

Figure 16.1 The NHS leadership qualities framework.

What is leadership?

> Leadership is different from management, but not for the reason people think. Leadership isn't mystical and mysterious. It has nothing to do with having charisma or other exotic personality traits. It's not the province of the chosen few. Nor is leadership necessarily better than management or a replacement for it: rather leadership and management are two distinctive and complementary activities. Both are necessary for success in an increasing complex and volatile business environment.[12]

Leadership is a complex social construct with 'almost as many definitions as there are persons who have attempted to define the concept',[13] and in recent years has attracted huge international interest. Leadership is increasingly seen as a panacea for the organisational ills of the twenty-first century and, as a result, there has been worldwide investment in leadership development. Even the NHS has developed its own leadership framework (Figure 16.1) and accompanying development programme.[14] But amidst this whirlwind of activity there remains no consensus as to what leadership is, in whom it resides and how best to develop leaders or leadership within an organisation. Perhaps as a consequence, there is little objective evidence as to whether it makes a difference on performance or productivity. Despite these misgivings, leadership is generally thought to be a good and necessary thing and, though elusive, continues to attract attention in organisations throughout both the private and public sectors.

> Leadership is like the Abominable Snowman, whose footprints are everywhere but who is nowhere to be seen.[15]

A recent review of the extensive leadership literature by Northhouse[16] identified four themes common to the various ways leadership has been conceived: namely, that leadership is a process, occurs in a group context and involves influence and goal attainment. The leadership literature from which these themes derive stretches back across the twentieth century and, to understand leadership better, it will help to examine the different lenses through which the concept has been viewed. What follows is a much abbreviated, potted, history.

In the first half of the century, leadership theory revolved around personal qualities. You either had these – usually in conjunction with a Y chromosome – or you did not. The so-called 'Great Man' theories emphasised characteristics such as intelligence, energy and dominance. However, several major reviews of the literature failed to consistently identify personality traits that differentiated leaders from non-leaders. Interestingly, trait theory has made a comeback in recent years with the emotional intelligence-based theories of Goleman and colleagues.[17]

From the 1950s onwards, attention shifted from personal characteristics of leaders to their behaviours. Blake and Mouton's[18] managerial grid is typical, plotting concern for the task and concern for people along the x and y axes, respectively (Figure 16.2). It was proposed that a high concern for both – 'team management' – was the most effective type of leadership behaviour.

Whilst these models introduced the idea of leadership as a group of behaviours, they gave little indication as to what sort of behaviours worked best in what circumstances. This was addressed through the work, among others, of Fiedler[19] and Hersey and Blanchard.[20] The latter achieved widespread popularity through the 'One-Minute Manager' series with their explication of 'situational leadership'. Hersey and Blanchard asserted that leaders needed to adapt their style to variations in the competence and commitment of followers. The four styles identified were directing, coaching, supporting and delegating (Figure 16.3).

A situational approach to leadership was also adopted by John Adair in his 'three circles model'.[21] Adair recommended that, depending on the circumstances, the focus of a leader's attention should be distributed flexibly between the task, the team and the individual (Figure 16.4).

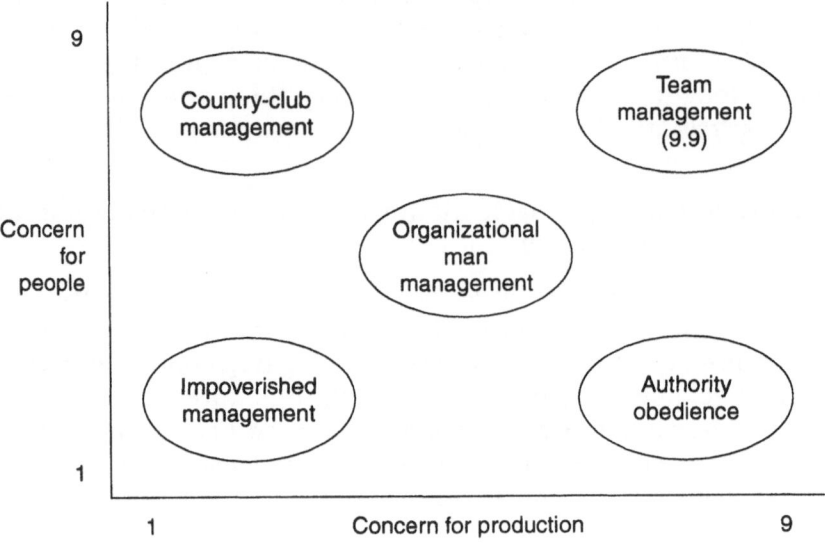

Figure 16.2 Behaviour-orientated leadership.[18]

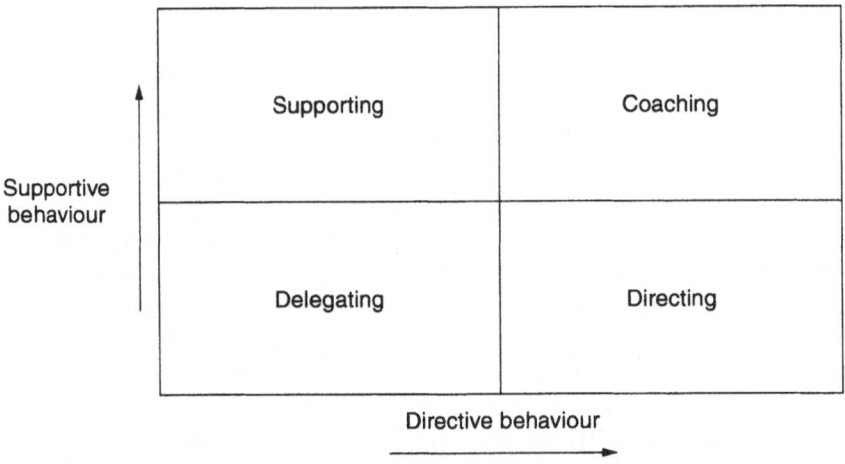

Figure 16.3 Situational leadership.[20]

It became apparent in the 1980s that none of the leadership theories to date offered advice on how to cope in environments of continuous change. Various authors highlighted that the models described so far were effectively managerial or transactional. They helped plan, order and organise at times of stability but were inadequate at describing how people or organisations might be led

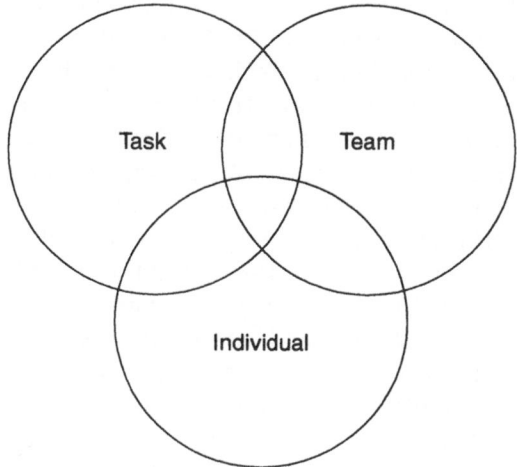

Figure 16.4 Action-centred leadership.[21]

through periods of significant change. A new paradigm emerged, that of 'trans-formational leadership' (Table 16.1), a concept best summarised under the four 'I's coined by Bass and Avolio,[22] namely:

- idealised influence
- inspirational motivation
- intellectual stimulation
- individual consideration.

Table 16.1 Transformational leadership[22]

Idealised influence
Moral, purposeful leadership through which is gained trust and respect
Transformational leaders behave in ways that result in their followers wishing to emulate them
Inspirational motivation
High expectations of commitment to a shared vision extending beyond the immediate concerns of followers, giving optimism, enthusiasm and meaning to the work of others
Intellectual stimulation
Innovation, problem-solving and creativity are encouraged and the status quo is constantly questioned
Individual consideration
A supportive climate is created in which individuals can address their own developmental needs; the transformational leader knows her staff well and encourages, rather than monitors, their efforts

In the transformational model, leaders act to release human potential through the empowerment and development of followers. Vision and values are clearly stated, and the organisation and the work of individuals within it are aligned to the achievement of longer-term goals. Transformational leadership has proved an enduring model and has been incorporated into many public-sector frameworks. Indeed, the influence of Bass and Avolio can be seen throughout our own NHS Leadership qualities framework (*see* Figure 16.1).

Before moving on to discussing how these theoretical notions of leadership and management can be acted on in the context of flexible training and working, one last theoretical strand is worthy of consideration. Known variously as 'informal', 'dispersed' or 'distributed leadership', this school of thought argues that no one individual is the ideal leader in all circumstances. It proposes that the locus of leadership is dissociated from the organisational hierarchy and that all members, not just those with an overt management function, can exert leadership influence over their colleagues. Leaders are emergent rather than predefined and their role is contingent on relationships rather than the characteristics of individuals. The model thus makes a key distinction between leaders and leadership in which organisations may be 'leaderless but leaderful'[23] or, indeed, vice versa.

Finally, a health warning. Although 'transactional' management and 'transformational' leadership have been represented as discrete entities, they are not. One cannot exist without the other and for individuals to manage effectively in organisations a balance is required. As Gosling and Mintzberg warn us:[24]

> The separation of management from leadership is dangerous. Just as management without leadership encourages an uninspired style, which deadens activities, leadership without management encourages a disconnected style, which promotes hubris. And we all know the destructive power of hubris in organizations.

Leadership, management and the doctor working flexibly

Doctors undertaking flexible training or working tend to have a number of characteristic features that will impact significantly on the nature and level of their engagement with management and leadership. 'Flexibles' are, by definition, part-time and the vast majority are women. They are employees, rather than employers, and have supernumerary status, which may be (wrongly) interpreted as superfluity.[25] Furthermore, doctors working flexibly may have centres of attention outside the organisation in which they work and a career which is often fractured and fragmentary. For a variety of reasons, then, ranging from a lack of opportunities to a loss of confidence, the default position for many flexible doctors is to adopt one of passive acquiescence. With a medical workforce that is increasingly becoming flexible, this will inevitably lead to increasing medical absenteeism from the tables of decision-making and direction-setting; an unsustainable situation in the long term.

Several of the issues discussed in this chapter are particularly pertinent to the doctor working flexibly, namely the role of doctors in leadership and management, where leadership is, or can be, sited in an organisation and issues of leadership and gender.

Doctors and management

Should doctors involve themselves in management? The answer must be 'yes'. Not only do doctors have the transferable skills of analysis, communication skills, problem-solving and decision-making, they have insider knowledge of the healthcare systems that require reform. Whether we like it or not, doctors are also looked to as leaders by other colleagues in the health service.

Healthcare improvement guru Donald Berwick makes the point that in improving systems we must concentrate on the needs of patients, not organisations.[26] Effective leaders, he says, challenge the status quo both by insisting that the current system cannot remain, and by offering clear ideas about superior alternatives. Meaningful system change can be brought about by constantly making small improvements. Doctors working flexibly are frequently marginal to the bureaucratic hierarchy of the healthcare organisation in which they work. This should not be a barrier to their involvement in service improvement. Patient-oriented incremental change is not dependent on an official management role, it is an activity with which all clinicians can engage.

Distributed leadership

Theories of distributed leadership propound that one does not have to occupy a leadership position to exert influence. In a complex world, coherence, making sense of things for others, is everyone's responsibility. Elsewhere in the public sector, most notably in education, this has led to the concept of the 'middle leader', with staff – often part-time, often female – in non-hierarchical management positions taking on leadership roles in specific areas of expertise.

A feminine future for leadership

Alimo-Metcalfe[27] has drawn our attention to the fact that leadership research has focused almost exclusively on white Western males in the top echelons of organisations. She argues that this gender-biased research has effectively theorised-out, or disenfranchised, vast populations at lower organisational levels and points to a growing body of evidence demonstrating the preference of many women leaders for transformational leadership. Such an approach, as we have seen, is strong on communication, building relationships and empowering others. In environments of high complexity and change, such as healthcare, it is also likely to be the approach required to achieve results. The research evidence is growing, but seems to indicate that women bring strengths to leadership and management that differ from, and may arguably be more effective than, those traditionally demonstrated by their male counterparts. Medical leadership positions to date have been dominated by men. In complex environments such as healthcare, the future of leadership may be feminine.

Conclusion

Leadership and management are complex, inter-related concepts essential for health service administration and reform. Both can be viewed as activities within organisations rather than as functions of specific job roles. Leadership and management are responsibilities of us all, and with an increasingly flexible workforce operating in an increasingly complex environment, this has never been more true. Sitting on the sidelines is not a sustainable option. In the words of the US advice columnist and epigrammatist, Ann Landers: 'There are really only three types of people: those who make things happen, those who watch things happen, and those who say, 'What happened?'''

References

1   Department of Health (2000) *The NHS Plan*. Department of Health, London.

2   Department of Health (2001) *Shifting the Balance of Power*. Department of Health, London.

3   Department of Health (2004) *NHS Improvement Plan*. Department of Health, London.

4   Department of Health (2005) *Commissioning a Patient-led NHS*. Department of Health, London.

5   The Institute of Public Health in Ireland (2004) *A Healthier Future: a twenty year vision for health and wellbeing in Northern Ireland 2005-2025*. Institute of Public Health, Ireland.

6   Scottish Executive (2000) *Our National Health: a plan for action, a plan for change*. Scottish Executive, Edinburgh.

7   Welsh Assembly (2001) *Improving Health in Wales: a plan for Wales*. Welsh Assembly, Cardiff.

8   Griffiths R (1983) *NHS Management Inquiry*. Department of Health and Social Security, London.

9   Simpson J (1994) Management for doctors: doctors and management – why bother? *BMJ*. **309**: 1505–1508.

10 Zaleznik A (1992) Managers and leaders: are they different? *Harvard Business Review*. **March**: 74–81.

11 Edwards N, Marshall M, McLellan A and Abbari K (2003) Doctors and managers: a problem without a solution? *BMJ*. **326**: 609–610.

12 Kotter JP (1990) What leaders really do. *Harvard Business Review*. **May–June**: 103–111.

13 Stodgill R (1974) *Handbook of Leadership: a survey of theory and research*. Free Press, New York.

14 NHS Leadership Centre (2003) *NHS Leadership Qualities Framework*. NHS Leadership Centre, London.

15 Bennis W and Nanus N (1985) *Leaders: strategies for taking charge*. Harper & Row, New York.

16 Northhouse P (2004) *Leadership: theory and practice* (3e). Sage, London.

17 Goleman D (2000) Leadership that gets results. *Harvard Business Review*. **March–April**: 78–90.

18 Blake R and Mouton J (1964) *The Managerial Grid*. Gulf, Houston.

19 Fiedler F (1964) A contingency model of leadership effectiveness. In: L Berkowitz (ed.) *Advances in Experimental Social Psychology*. Academic Press, New York.

20 Hersey P and Blanchard K (1988) *Management of Organizational Behaviour*. Prentice Hall, Englewood Cliffs.

21 Adair J (1973) *Action-centred Leadership*. McGraw-Hill, New York.

22 Bass B and Avolio B (1994) *Improving Organizational Effectiveness Through Transformational Leadership*. Sage, Thousand Oaks.

23 Vanderslice V (1988) Separating leadership from leaders: an assessment of the effect of leader and follower roles. *Human Relations*. **41**: 677–696.

24 Gosling J and Mintzberg H (2003) The five minds of a manager. *Harvard Business Review*. **November**: 54-63.

25 Swanwick T and Plint S (2006) From supernumerary to supervised professional development. *Education for General Practice*. **17**: 97–103.

26 Berwick D (1996) A primer on the improvement of systems. *BMJ*. **312**: 619–622.

27 Alimo-Metcalfe B (2002) *Leadership and Gender: a masculine past; a feminine future*. University of Leeds, Leeds.

CHAPTER 17

Illness and disability

Antony Americano

Introduction

Organisational policies often afford ill and disabled people priority consideration when they ask to work and train flexibly. Despite this positive approach by
educational managers and employers, the day-to-day handling of requests can
be unsatisfactory on both sides. Barriers, both organisational and attitudinal,
which exist towards flexible training are compounded with concerns raised by
ill health and disability. Concerns may legitimately raise patient safety and
health and safety risks but fail to take into account other legal responsibilities.
A solution-focused approach is required.

This chapter aims to assist in managing requests for flexibility from ill and
disabled people in a way that is sensitive to the needs of the individuals and the
organisation. By understanding the differing conceptualisations of disability, the
legal framework, current terminology and how to manage reasonable adjustments, an approach will be encouraged that increases the chances of positive
individual and organisational outcomes. Learning tasks will be used throughout the chapter to help further understanding, and additional resources are
highlighted to assist further study. The approach to disability used will be based
on a social rather than a medical model, which may require clinical staff to
adjust their cognitive framework.

What is disability?

Legal dimension

Although legislation on disability has been on the statutes for many years, it is
the last decade that has seen significant developments. Legislation has been
enacted and amended, statutory bodies have been created and codes of practice
written (Box 17.1). The overall effect has been to increase the legal rights of
disabled people and to give educational bodies and employers responsibilities
to respond positively and pro-actively to disabled students and workers.

Box 17.1 Legal framework for disability

Disability Discrimination Act 1995
This Act has progressively made it illegal to treat disabled people less favourably in employment, in the provision of goods, facilities and services, and in education. Education has been covered by the Act since September 2002 and requires schools, colleges, universities and providers of adult education and youth services to ensure that they do not discriminate against disabled people. In October 2004, the Act was further extended to cover organisations that confer, renew or extend a professional or trade qualification. It is therefore unlawful for a qualifications body to discriminate against a disabled person when awarding, renewing, extending or withdrawing a professional or trade qualification.

Disability Rights Commission Act 1999
The legislation which established the Disability Rights Commission (DRC) in April 2000 with statutory duties to eliminate discrimination, promote equal opportunities and encourage good practice and treatment of disabled people. Their website is a useful source of information (www.drc-gb.org.uk).

Codes of practice
The DRC has established a number of codes of practice. These do not have the authority of law but can be considered by courts when assessing the appropriateness of an employer's behaviour. There are codes covering, among other things, employment, responsibility of qualification bodies and guidance for providers of post-16 education. These are essential reading given their influence on legal decisions.

Special Educational Needs and Disability Act 2001
This Act gives the right for disabled students not to be discriminated against in education, training and any services provided wholly or mainly for students, and this includes higher education. It does this through a series of amendments to the Disability Discrimination Act. A wide range of educational and non-educational services are covered, for example field trips, examinations and assessments, short courses, arrangements for work placements and libraries and learning resources.

Medical Act 1983
The Act provides a mechanism for the General Medical Council (GMC) to approve training programmes for disabled students who are not able to meet the current experiential legislative requirements. The requirements of the DDA will mean that outcome measures will need to be considered more than input.

How does the Disability Discrimination Act define disability?

- It can be a physical or mental impairment.
- It must have a substantial effect, which somewhat unhelpfully is defined as being 'more than just minor or trivial'.
- That effect must be on a person's ability to carry out day-to-day tasks. This phrase refers to tasks that a typical person undertakes and not work-related tasks.
- The disability must also have lasted at least 12 months or be expected to do so. This can include conditions that are expected to reoccur beyond the 12-month period. Individuals who have recovered or are in remission from conditions such as cancer are also protected from discrimination.

This is a broad definition that initially raised more questions than answers. Developing case law has led to greater understanding of its interpretation. A recent example involved an individual with Asperger syndrome, in which the ability to participate in human interactions, social relationships and communications was considered to be a day-to-day activity. Accordingly, the requirement for the employer to consider reasonable adjustments was triggered.[1] Cases in progress, supported by the DRC, include students with dyslexia and with Asperger syndrome who have been refused entry into university nursing degree courses.[2] Barriers to disabled people's participation in education are still very real.

Amendments to the Disability Discrimination Act have extended its protection. Although previously mental impairments had to be clinically well recognised, this is no longer the case. Additionally, individuals are deemed to be disabled at the point of diagnosis for conditions such as HIV, multiple sclerosis and cancer even if the condition does not have substantial effect on their ability to carry out day-to-day activities.

The Act also requires employers and service providers to make 'reasonable adjustments' to assist disabled people in the workplace and in accessing services. This topic will be explored in some detail later on in the chapter.

Learning task 1

Below is a list of conditions. Consider whether you think these should be considered as disabilities under the Disability Discrimination Act. Answers are at the end of this chapter.

- alcoholism
- anxiety/depression
- asthma/diabetes well controlled by medication
- claustrophobia
- inability to undertake activities requiring delicate hand movements such as threading a small needle
- taking significantly longer than average to say something
- urinary incontinence resulting from prostate cancer

Models of disability

Your approach to illness and disability will probably depend on your exposure to differing models of disability. What are these? A good example of one model is an early definition of disability developed for the World Health Organization (WHO):

> Any restriction or lack (resulting from an impairment) of ability to perform an activity in the manner or within the range considered normal for a human being.[3]

This definition angered many disability rights supporters with its basis in the medical model of disability (*see* Table 17.1). Barnes *et al.* (1999) criticised the work of the WHO because it attempted to define 'normal', ignored environmental factors and was focused on a cure.[4]

Another approach has been defined as the charitable model of disability (*see* Table 17.1). In this model, the disabled person is seen as a tragic individual who needs help to cope with their loss. This leads to one of two scenarios: either disabled people are seen as objects of pity who need to be cared for and protected from the demands of daily life or some individuals may be held up as 'heroes' who have bravely triumphed over adversity. These 'heroes' are special and not an example of what can be achieved by disabled people generally.

Table 17.1 Differences between models of disability

	Medical model	Charitable model	Social model
The individual	Individual is a patient or dependent	Individual is a charity case or hero (dependent or exceptional)	Individual is a distinct member of society with rights and is independent
Source of problem	Medical condition	Impairment	Attitudes in and organisation of society
Solution/ approach	Medical intervention/ conditions to be treated/controlled	Provide help; case to be pitied/made heroic	Change society, ensure individuals' rights
Locus of power	Responsibility held by clinical staff	Responsibility held by 'charitable' staff or volunteers	Responsibility held by disabled people

Organisations representing disabled people have proposed very different definitions. The Union of Physically Impaired Against Segregation (UPIAS) defined disability as:

> The disadvantage or restriction caused by a contemporary social organisation which takes no or little account of people who have physical impairments and thus excludes them from the mainstream of social activities.[5]

Therefore people with impairments are disabled not by physical impairments but by attitudes and barriers in society. In practice the social model of disability, which has its roots in the work of UPIAS, suggests that rather than considering the seriousness of individuals' impairments we should consider the level of adjustment that is required to surmount societal barriers. Effectively, this alters our approach from measuring a problem to seeking a solution in partnership with the disabled person.

Because of the remit of UPIAS, the definition only covered physical disability. Nevertheless, this definition represented a major reconceptualisation of disability which was later built upon by Michael Oliver. The social model has been much developed and analysed over the last 30 years. It has also been critiqued in academic circles but such analysis is beyond the scope of this chapter. Table 17.1 summarises the major differences between models.

Learning task 2
Choose a clinical activity and consider what the attitudinal, organisational and physical barriers there might be for various forms of impairment. How difficult or easy would it be to surmount these? Whose support would you need?

Caring for disabled dependants

In some cases, the person wishing to work or train flexibly will wish to do so because of a dependant's illness or disability rather than their own. Where the dependant is a child, the law confers particular rights.

Part-time workers regulations

The legal right to request flexible working, which covers children under the age of six years, and increases to 18 for disabled children. The request can cover hours of work, times of work and place of work, and can involve requests for different patterns of work, including:

- flexi-time
- home working
- term-time working
- shift working
- self-rostering
- annualised hours.

The request must be made in writing and the employer has a statutory duty to consider the request seriously and to refuse it only if there are clear grounds for so doing. The nature of medicine and dentistry will provide a case for refusing some, but by no means all, patterns of work, and each case must be considered individually, taking into account the individual's needs (including the level and type of care the disabled child needs), the specific staffing situation (numbers, other part-timers) and the demands of their particular branch of medicine or dentistry, including, of course, the issue of patient safety. Individuals making applications for flexible working have the right to be accompanied at meetings by a fellow employee.

Parental leave regulations

Staff who have one year's service with their employer are entitled to 13 weeks' unpaid parental leave for each child born or adopted. The leave can start once the child is born or placed for adoption or as soon as the individual has completed a year's service, whichever is later. It may be taken at any time up to the child's fifth birthday (or until five years after placement in the case of adoption). Parents of disabled children can take 18 weeks up to the child's 18th birthday.

Time off for dependants

All employees are entitled to a reasonable time off work without pay, to deal with an emergency involving a dependant. For example, if a dependant falls ill or is injured, if care arrangements break down or have to be set up, or to arrange or attend a dependant's funeral. It cannot be used to manage ongoing care needs.

Illness and disability: myths and misconceptions

When does an illness become a disability? The legal definition of disability is explained above but the division between them is socially constructed and subject to change as society's views and available technology evolve. Because of the legal protection now afforded to disabled people, much time can be spent deciding whether an illness constitutes a legal disability. However, attempts to second-guess the courts are rarely fruitful. For a whole host of legal and best-practice reasons, the better approach is to deal with each situation with an open mind and a desire to end exclusion for ill and disabled members of society. Additionally, skilled staff should be supported to remain in the NHS workforce wherever reasonably possible.

You will not be alone if you have only a vague understanding of disability. For example, although wheelchair users represent only about 5% of those with impairments, they are, nevertheless, the image most associated with 'disability'. Unseen impairments, such as asthma, epilepsy and diabetes, are often forgotten or misunderstood. Mental health and learning difficulties raise prejudices and fears with significant misconceptions, for example, about conditions such as autism and dyslexia (*see* Box 17.2).

Box 17.2 Common myths about disability

Equal opportunities means we should treat disabled people the same as others

Equal opportunities is about giving everyone an equal chance to advance their medical and dental career, develop skills, etc. If you do not remove barriers they cannot have an equal chance.

Adjustments for disabled people are prohibitively expensive

Many reasonable adjustments may not cost anything but simply require the organisation to do things differently. Where there are costs, many adjustments are a matter of few hundred pounds and government financial support is available for higher costs.

Disabled people will take up too much staff/manager time

If they obtained a medical or dental degree, it is already clear that the individual is strongly motivated to, and experienced in, overcoming barriers. If they have recently acquired an impairment, the input required will be worthwhile to safeguard the considerable investment in their education already made.

Other myths

- Disability is a monumental tragedy/disabled people are brave and saintly.
- Disabled people who do 'normal' things are exceptional.
- Disabled people lead boring and uneventful lives/are asexual.

Disability is complex and not all people with an impairment experience it in the same way. Treat people as individuals, ask their opinion and seek advice where appropriate. An example of this complexity is that the word 'Deaf', when used with a capital 'D', refers to people who belong to the Deaf community. Many Deaf community members do not see themselves as disabled people but as members of a cultural and linguistic minority community who use sign language as their first language.

Exploring further, we learn that there is more than one type of sign language. There is British Sign Language (BSL), Makaton, deaf manual, blind manual and more. It is important to remember that a person using one form of sign language may not know others. When arranging sign language interpretations you must ensure you provide the sign language the person uses. To complicate matters further, remember that not all deaf or hearing-impaired people use sign language.

Learning task 3
Select an impairment with which you are unfamiliar. Use the Additional Resources below to learn more about the impairment, going beyond clinical information. Reflect on how your previous understanding of the impairment was formed and how your new understanding differs.

Terminology

Thoughtful use of language is important in showing respect and empowering individuals. Most people do not like being referred to by medical labels: 'asthmatics', 'schizophrenics', but may find the term 'people with asthma', etc., more acceptable. 'Handicapped' has cap-in-hand associations with charity and is largely out of favour. However, there are considerable differences between groups and individuals as to how they prefer to be addressed. A general guide follows in Table 17.2 but it is always best to ask individuals about their preferences.

Table 17.2 Advice on terminology

Avoid	Use
The disabled	Disabled people
Able-bodied, healthy, normal	Non-disabled, person without a disability
Handicapped/cripple/invalid	Disabled person
Victim of/suffering from . . .	Person who has/person with . . .
Wheelchair-bound	Wheelchair user
Epileptic/asthmatic/arthritic/ diabetic/dyslexic/schizophrenic	Person who has/person with . . .
The blind	People with a visual impairment
The deaf	People with a hearing impairment
Mute	Speech or communication disability
Spastic	Person with cerebral palsy
Mental handicap/retard	Person with a learning difficulty
Person who is mad/mental/crazy	Person with mental health difficulties/problems

In general, you should not try to alter standard speech, for example 'Did you hear?' rather than 'Did you see?' a film. Most disabled people are not worried about such language. Even if you say something in the wrong way, simply apologise, maintain a sense of humour and keep communicating rather than withdrawing.

Barriers in society and in medicine and dentistry

The 2001 Census indicated that there were 6.8 million people of working age who can be classified as having a long-term impairment.[6] This equates to nearly one in five people. How does this translate into the workplace? Disabled people had an employment rate of 48% compared to a figure of 81% for non-disabled people.[7] Impairments are therefore a major barrier to participation at work.

Turning to education: in 2000, disabled students represented only 4% of applicants to university and this figure rose to 5% by 2004. Accepted applicants broadly reflected the numbers applying. The impairments disclosed are mostly in the areas of dyslexia and unseen conditions such as asthma and diabetes,[8] Generally, disabled people are less likely to have academic or vocational qualifications.[9] This is a significant barrier to entry into medicine and dentistry and professions allied to medicine. Disabled applicants made up 2% of applicants for medicine in 2000 and just under 3% of applicants in 2003.[10] Those disabled doctors and dentists that do exist often acquired an impairment during their studies or whilst working, therefore avoiding the barriers of entry to medical/dental school.

There has been a steadily growing recognition of these issues in medicine and dentistry. In 2001, disability was highlighted when Heidi Cox, a disabled applicant to medical school took the GMC to an employment tribunal for discrimination. The applicant had been offered a place but required modifications to the course.[10] The GMC said that it could not alter the curriculum but was criticised by the employment tribunal. Although, at the time, the GMC successfully appealed against the negative findings, the case emphasised that disabled people encounter significant barriers to becoming doctors.

A few years later, the British Medical Association (BMA) published a report on career barriers in medicine. This identified in some detail that disabled doctors continued to face significant discrimination and concluded that this problem required urgent action.[11]

The GMC *Good Medical Practice*[12] sets out the following standards for doctors:

There should be support for students and doctors who wish to learn and work flexibly. Reasonable adjustments should be made for those students and doctors who have a disability. Students and doctors with a wide range of disabilities or health conditions will often be able to achieve the standards set for knowledge, skills, attitudes and behaviours.

This sets the scene for the consideration of reasonable adjustments which follows.

Reasonable adjustments

Introduction

The Disability Discrimination Act requires employers and training bodies to consider and implement reasonable adjustments. If a disabled person is at a 'substantial disadvantage', responsible bodies are required to take reasonable steps to prevent that disadvantage. These might include:

- making changes to policies and practices
- changes to the physical features of a building
- provision of interpreters or other support workers
- delivery of courses in alternative ways
- provision of material in other formats
- provide (re)training
- 'partnering' with a non-disabled person or mentor
- alter work/workplace by redesigning duties
- provision of special equipment.

Disabled people tend to be the experts in how to manage their own impairment so a constructive dialogue is the best approach to identifying reasonable adjustments. If an individual trainee/employee is not sure of the solution, it may be that another disabled trainee or member of staff has relevant experience that can be shared. There are also a number of agencies set up by disabled people to provide consultancy advice on access/adaptation issues (*see* Additional Resources).

When is an adjustment reasonable?

This is a complex question and depends on a number of factors:

- size and resources of the organisation (e.g. a large acute hospital trust may be expected to do more than a small GP practice)
- cost of the adjustment
- amount already spent on such adjustments
- whether the adjustment will make a significant difference to the disabled person.

Although the Act does not mention them, other factors, such as the effect on other employees, adjustments made for other disabled employees and the extent to which the disabled person is willing to co-operate, may be relevant.

Offering flexible working constitutes a reasonable adjustment. However, although some disabled people may request this, it should not be assumed that the majority would always prefer this option. Disabled people are usually not ill and are often comfortable with their impairment. The ability to work full-time can be important for social inclusion giving them, among other things, a reasonable living wage to pursue interests. Consequently, allowing barriers to prevent this is detrimental to the individual, damaging to the workforce and open to legal challenge.

Types of barriers faced by disabled people

Where flexible training is a reasonable adjustment and one requested by the disabled person there are three main types of barriers.

Attitudinal barriers

The team that the individual will have to work in may have prejudices and fears about working with someone with an impairment. This may lead to hostility, a patronising approach, marginalisation or generally less favourable treatment. The team members may not be conscious of their attitude and may even be attempting to help by, for example, keeping the disabled person away from 'difficult' work. Providing information, support and disability awareness training to the team in order to understand the barriers that inhibit the disabled person will help avoid these situations. Issues to address include:

- cost to the employer – will this be to the detriment of the service to patients?
- negative impact on colleagues' morale, performance or workloads
- need for increased supervision
- increased risk of accidents
- uncertainty about absences for health reasons.

Patients may also feel uncomfortable and question the competence of the doctor or dentist, based solely on their impairment. It is important to consider how to address such issues as they arise. This is naturally a difficult process with patient rights possibly conflicting with individual rights. Nevertheless, it is important not to collude with discrimination.

Institutional and organisational barriers

These can include scheduling of work hours and rota systems. Time-related problems, such as long intervals between mealtimes or limited opportunities to visit lavatories or bathrooms, may also cause difficulties. It is also important to review policies in force (e.g. allowing guide dogs as an exception to a 'no dogs' rule) to ensure that they do not discriminate unreasonably.

Physical barriers

These are usually associated with mobility-related impairments, in particular with people who are wheelchair users. Indeed, building design is an important cause of disability. However, physical barriers also include:

- difficulties with the legibility or comprehensible nature of the printed word, for example preparing all handouts using at least 12 point Arial or other sans serif font printed on yellow or buff coloured paper will help dyslexic students, but also make them more readable for all students
- poorly visible or inadequately lit locations
- weak colour contrast or excessive complexity in text or diagrams and maps
- lack of signers or induction loops
- poorly designed screen displays in software or presentations.

Type and location of equipment should be considered to ensure that they are usable by all. Health and safety procedures should consider all staff, for example the provision of a visual signal with a fire alarm.

Learning task 4
Consider the barriers in your workplace under the three headings above. What actions could be taken immediately to address them?

Health and safety concerns

The GMC position on the viability of adjustments is that the safety of the public must always come first. Indeed, case law confirms that health and safety issues, including those relating to the individual and colleagues, are valid defences when considering the requirements of the Disability Discrimination Act provided appropriate adjustments/measures have first been considered.[13] Fitness to practise procedures will need to be evoked where appropriate. Nevertheless, to stay within the law, educational bodies and employers will need to show they are actively supporting disabled people to achieve full participation in society, as the GMC Education Committee notes in relation to pre-registration house officers (PRHOs):

> All PRHOs, including those with a wide range of disabilities and health conditions, can achieve full registration provided that they meet all the outcomes. However, each individual's situation is different and therefore has to be considered individually by those responsible for training, in conjunction with the employing Trusts. Additional support and training must be provided for any PRHO who has been unable to complete training because of ill health or disability.[14]

If patient safety or health and safety concerns are to be raised, and of course this is quite legitimate and necessary, it is important to consider objectively whether requirements or competencies are proportionate to achieving their aims and whether alternatives or reasonable adjustments could remove or diminish the risk. These assessments should be completed for each individual case and not in a blanket fashion covering a particular impairment. The Health and Safety Executive has produced research suggesting that health and safety reasons are too readily used as an excuse to discriminate against disabled people.[15]

Answers to learning task 1
Please note that decisions in legal cases can turn on facts peculiar to themselves and that case law is continuously developing. The information below should not be considered a definitive statement of the law.

- Alcoholism is specifically excluded from the Disability Discrimination Act but conditions resulting from abuse of alcohol may themselves be covered.
- Anxiety/depression – these may be considered disabilities under the Act but it would depend on individual circumstances. It is sensible to approach staff with these conditions as if they were disabled.
- Asthma/diabetes – the law states that in assessing whether someone is disabled it is necessary to look at the impact of the condition pre-treatment.
- Claustrophobia can be considered as a disability according to case law.
- Inability to undertake delicate hand movements would not normally be covered under the Act as these would not be considered to be day-to-day activities. The inability to handle a knife and fork would very likely be considered a disability.
- Taking significantly longer to articulate would be considered a disability. Minor lisps or stutters would probably not but a significant speech impediment would.
- Urinary incontinence was considered by a court to be part of the progressive condition of prostate cancer. In particular, it was noted that this was a common outcome from a surgical procedure which is regularly carried out in response to this condition.

Summary

There are clear and unavoidable responsibilities for employers and educators to provide an environment where disabled people can participate fully in medicine and dentistry. The gains if this is achieved are significant, including the social inclusion of a group of people experiencing widespread discrimination and organisational benefits such as the retention of skilled staff and the creation of a diverse workforce with first-hand experience of impairment. Provision of flexibility of hours, geography and content is important, but it is only one of a number of reasonable adjustments which may be needed to create a level playing field.

Further information

The following lists are some examples of useful resources but they are by no means comprehensive. Links were confirmed as active at time of writing.

Agencies

- Disability Matters (www.disabilitymatters.com)

Carers

- Employers for Carers (www.employersforcarers.org.uk)
- CarersUK (www.carersuk.org)

Education and employment

- Disability and Learning and Teaching: Disability Discrimination Act – pre-sessional advice for teaching staff. (www.lancs.ac.uk)
- Skill: National bureau for students with disabilities. Skill is a national charity promoting opportunities for young people and adults with any kind of disability in post-16 education, training and employment across the UK. (www.skill.org.uk)
- Disability Rights Commission: there are employment and education microsites with useful information. You can also become licensed to use their training pack. (www.drc.org.uk)
- Employers' Forum on Disability: Network of major employers working to provide employment for disabled people. (www.employers-forum.co.uk/www/index.htm)
- Employment Services: Government support for disabled people at work. (www.direct.gov.uk/DisabledPeople/Employment/fs/en)

Reasonable adjustments

- Centre for Accessible Environments: provides information, design guidance, training and consultancy services. (www.cae.org.uk)
- Ability Net: offers a 'one-stop-shop' for all your assistive technology needs. (www.abilitynet.co.uk)
- British Educational Communications and Technology Agency: BECTA is the government's key partner in the strategic development and delivery of its information and communications technology (ICT) and e-learning strategy for schools and the learning and skills sectors. (www.becta.org.uk)
- Communications Matters: a UK national charitable organisation of members concerned with the augmentative and alternative communication (AAC) needs of people with complex communication needs. (www.communicationmatters.org.uk)
- Limbless Association: helps limbless people of all ages (and their carers) achieve maximum mobility and independence in home, hospital, education, employment and the community. (www.limbless-association.org)

Specific impairments

- University of Gloucestershire: information on how to treat people who are wheelchair users. (www2.glos.ac.uk/gdn/disability/mobility/protocol.htm)
- Radar: has an excellent links section about specific impairments. (www.radar.org.uk/Links/Linksgraphics.asp)

References

1 Industrial Relations Law Review (2004) Hewett v Motorola Ltd. *IRLR.* **545**: EAT.

2 Disability Rights Commission. (www.drc-gb.org/drc/InformationAndLegislation/Page356.asp (Accessed October 2005)

3 Wood P (1980) *International Classification of Impairments, Disabilities and Handicaps.* World Health Organization, Geneva.

4 Barnes C, Mercer G and Shakespeare T (1999) *Exploring Disability: a sociological introduction.* Blackwell, Oxford.

5 Disability Awareness in Action: the international disability and human rights network. (www.daa.org.uk/social_model.html) (Accessed August 2005)

6 Office of National Statistics (2001) Economic activity status of disabled people: by gender. *Social Trends.* **32**. (www.statistics.gov.uk/census) (Accessed October 2005)

7 Smith A and Twomey B (2002). Labour market experiences of people with disabilities. *Labour Market Trends.* **110**: 415–27.

8 Universities and Colleges Clearing Service. (www.ucas.com/figures/ucasdata/disability/index.html) (Accessed September 2005)

9   Hurstfield *et al.* (2004) *Qualifications Bodies and the Disability Discrimination Act.* Report 417, Institute for Employment Studies, London.

10 Disability Rights Commission. Website: General Medical Council v Heidi Cox (EAT/76/01). (www.drc.org.uk/thelaw)

11 British Medical Association (2004) *Career Barriers in Medicine: doctors' experiences.* BMA, London.

12 General Medical Council (2001) *Good Medical Practice.* GMC, London.

13 Employment Appeals Tribunal. Website: Lane Group PLC vs. Farmiloe (2004) UK EAT/0352/ 03 (www.employmentappeals.gov.uk/judge_fr.htm) (Accessed October 2005)

14 General Medical Council (2004) Education Committee 22 July 2004 *Item B: The Review of PRHO Training Seminar on Disability: 18 June 2004.* (www.gmc.org.uk)

15 Health and Safety Executive (2003) *The Extent to Use Health and Safety Requirements as a False Excuse for Not Employing Sick or Disabled Persons.* HSE research report 167. (www.hse.gov.uk) (Accessed October 2005)

CHAPTER 18

Pensions, maternity leave and other benefits

Anne Hastie

Introduction

The National Health Service (NHS) provides doctors and dentists with very good benefits under the General Whitley Council Conditions of Service.[1] Dental and medical practitioners working in primary care within the NHS (NHS practitioners) also have access to benefits, although there are some differences. It is particularly important that doctors and dentists who are working flexibly or part-time, or both, are aware of the rules and regulations of NHS benefits to help them plan their future.

During the First World War a committee was convened by the Rt Hon J H Whitley MP to write a report on the improvement in the relations between employers and their employees. The committee's final report established a Civil Service National Whitley Council that determined the conditions of service.[2] In 1948 the NHS was introduced, which adopted the principles and practices of the Whitley Council. There was a Whitley Council for each staff group in the NHS, including doctors and dentists.[3]

Under the government's new *Agenda for Change* the Whitley Council was replaced by new NHS terms of service for NHS staff in the *Agenda for Change* handbook, except for doctors and dentists who continued with their Whitley Council terms and conditions of service. The conditions are regularly updated and further changes are inevitable, as the Department of Health would like all doctors and dentists to also be covered by the *Agenda for Change* handbook.

Pensions

The NHS pension scheme has many benefits, which are protected. Recent pension difficulties for workers in the private sector or those with personal pensions have highlighted the advantages of public-sector pensions. No one is too young to be thinking about a pension, and the earlier a pension is started the better the benefits on retirement. Doctors and dentists are recommended to stay in the NHS pension scheme and the few who have opted out have often regretted their decision. Actuaries have assessed the benefits of the NHS pension scheme as being worth approximately 20% of overall pay.[4] The following information is a summary of the main points of the NHS pension scheme but doctors and dentists are advised to seek professional advice on an individual basis.

Benefits of the NHS pension scheme include:

- tax-free lump sum
- index-linked pension, in line with the cost of living
- life assurance while working, which includes a tax-free lump sum, spouse pension and child allowance
- enhanced pension as a result of redundancy
- enhanced pension as a result of ill health retirement.

Doctors and dentists, except NHS practitioners, currently (2006) have their pensions based on the best of their last three years' pay. Forty years' membership of the scheme at the age of 60 years provides a full NHS pension. The NHS pension scheme is currently (2006) undergoing a strategic review and up to date information is available from the NHS Pension Agency (www.nhspa.gov.uk) and the British Medical Association (BMA) (www.bma.org.uk).

The main issues that are under review are:

- normal pension age raised to 65 years
- final-salary pension changed to career-average pension
- purchasing added years may not exist in a new scheme
- partners' pension to include unmarried and same-sex partners
- choice of lump sum
- new arrangements to apply to new members.

Retirement age

The current (2006) retirement age in the NHS is 60 years and the overall limit on the NHS pension scheme is 45 years. Membership can continue until 70 years, although this may alter with new legislation on age discrimination. Early retirement can be taken voluntarily from age 50 years with an actuarial reduction, which is age-related. Members who have worked part-time have their membership and final year's pay changed to the equivalent full-time amount, which is then used to work out the member's pension. Doctors can return to work after retirement following a break of one month, although they cannot rejoin the NHS pension scheme after retirement.

Doctors with mental health officer (MHO) status before 6 March 1995 can retire with benefits from 55 years if they have at least 20 years working as an MHO. Each year of MHO membership over 20 years counts as two years for benefit purposes.

The government's review on public-sector pensions proposed a change in retirement age from 60 to 65 years for new entrants, with protection to existing members until 2013. This has been strongly opposed by the BMA, which wants protection for all existing members.

Pensions for practitioners

NHS practitioners, including GPs providing general medical services (GMS), personal medical services (PMS) and dentists providing general dental services (GDS), are pensioned under the practitioner method, which is based on career-average earnings. The pensionable pay for each year of membership is uprated to the pay levels in force when the practitioner stops paying contributions and this is known as 'dynamising'. Since 1 April 2004 pension contributions are assessed on actual GP pensionable earnings declared to the Inland Revenue and are based on NHS profit net of expenses. The current NHS pension review is suggesting the career-average method of calculating pensions should be used for all doctors and dentists.

If a practitioner has some hospital or other NHS officer membership the Pensions Agency will automatically assess whether it is possible and beneficial to convert to a practitioner pension for all work or give a separate pension for the officer work. Practitioner membership cannot be converted to a final salary pension and the rules are complex (*see* www.nhspa.gov.uk).

GPs working as locums can pay contributions to the NHS pension scheme on their gross pay less 10% for expenses, and membership of the scheme is built up in the same way as salaried GPs. The locum must be deputising for a NHS GP, NHS GP practice or out-of-hours GP, all of whom must be registered with the NHS pension scheme. Locums forward contributions to their primary care trust (PCT) on a monthly basis with the relevant GP locum contribution forms. There is a time limit for GP locum contributions of 10 weeks from the end of any period of locum work.

Ill health retirement

Retirement on health grounds while still in NHS pensionable employment may result in additional membership of the NHS pension scheme. If a member has between five and 10 years of pensionable NHS employment the membership is doubled. If membership is more than 10 years it is either increased to 20 years up to a maximum age of 65 years or increased by 6.66 years subject to the maximum achievable membership by 60 years. The member will receive the most beneficial method but the total length of membership cannot be more than 40 years. Alternatively, if a member is seriously ill and not expected to live longer than one year they may apply for a bigger lump sum.

Additional pension options

Being a member of the NHS pension scheme allows other means of increasing income at retirement:

- Purchasing guaranteed additional years of service.
- Additional voluntary contributions (AVCs) are an arrangement with external insurance companies selected by the NHS Pension Agency.
- Free Standing additional voluntary contributions (FSAVCs) can be purchased from any insurance company.
- A stakeholder pension can be taken out with contributions of up to £3600 per year for five years providing the individual's pay is less than £30,000 in the first year.
- If a doctor or dentist has paid enough National Insurance contributions they will be entitled to a state pension, which would normally be the flat rate retirement pension.
- From April 2006 new government arrangements for pensions taxation will allow more flexibility for doctors and dentists to make contributions to personal pensions in addition to the NHS pension scheme.
- There will be a cap on total lifetime pension savings, which will be £1.5 million for 2006/2007 and may affect high-earning doctors and dentists.
- Other savings in cash or equities, such as Individual Savings Accounts (ISAs).

Life assurance and family benefits

If a doctor or dentist dies during NHS pensionable employment a tax-free lump sum is payable equal to two years' pensionable pay and the spouse gets a pension based on length of service. For NHS practitioners, the lump sum is twice the annual average of the total uprated pensionable pay. However, GP locums only have partial death in service benefits and this is currently being disputed by the BMA. If death occurs after retirement the spouse gets a pension equal to half the full pension, although this may be smaller if the marriage occurred after retirement. There are also allowances for dependent children but the amount of benefits will depend on the length of service and individual circumstances. However, a widower only gets half the pension his wife would have received from any membership of the scheme after 6 April 1988.

Redundancy

Redundancy, although rare for doctors and dentists, may occur as a result of organisational restructuring, closure of a NHS unit or reduction of workload. There is a possibility that redundancy may become more common as other providers take over work from the NHS. In such circumstances the employer should consider alternative employment and if this is not possible staff may be offered voluntary redundancy or voluntary early retirement. Compulsory redundancy should be the last alternative and there is an appeals process.

Redundancy payments are calculated on age and length of service. If a doctor or dentist is aged over 50 years and has at least five years in the NHS pension scheme an enhanced pension and lump sum may be payable. The maximum enhanced pension is 10 years to a maximum age of 65 years, or 40 years of service. An enhanced pension is not available to GPs because there is no employer to pay the extra costs involved. In all situations doctors and dentists should seek advice from their relevant trade union, such as the BMA.

Sickness benefits

The NHS has legal responsibilities under health and safety legislation, and has taken an increasing interest in preventing and supporting health problems in staff. Doctors and dentists have access to confidential occupational health services whose main function is to try and prevent ill health and accidents at work.

Allowances during sick leave

NHS employed doctors and dentists who become absent from duty owing to illness, injury or other disability receive the following sick leave allowances.

- During the first year of service: one month of full pay and after completing four months of service two months at half pay.
- During the second year of service: two months of full pay followed by two months of half pay.
- During the third year of service: four months of full pay followed by four months of half pay.
- During the fourth and fifth years of service: five months of full pay followed by five months of half pay.
- After completing five years service: six months of full pay followed by six months of half pay.

Where statutory sick pay and other benefits are added to the sickness allowance the total payment must not exceed the individual's normal salary and consequently the sick leave allowance is reduced by the amount of other payments.

Sickness benefits for GPs

The PCT may pay a contribution to the practice towards the cost of a locum when a GP performer takes sick leave and a locum is employed. The regulations are complex[5] and the PCT can use discretion over payments. In accordance with the BMA model contract for salaried GPs the practitioner on sick leave should be entitled to receive the allowances described above from their employing practice. All previous NHS service (including locum service) is aggregated for the purposes of sick leave and there are specific circumstances in which a break of more than 12 months' service does not mean a break in qualifying service. The rights of GP partners to paid sickness leave are a matter for their partnership agreement. All GPs, whether employed or in partnership, are advised to ensure their contract adequately covers sick leave.

Maternity and adoption leave

Maternity leave legislation was amended as a result of the Employment Act 2003 and implemented from 6 April 2003.[6] Most NHS medical staff are covered by the General Whitley Council agreement, which is more generous than statutory employment law.[7] GP registrars are employed by their GP practice and not the NHS but there is an agreement that they are entitled to similar maternity leave and pay as the Whitley agreement. Salaried GPs should ensure their contract has a continuity clause to cover previous NHS work before joining their current practice. The regulations are complex and individuals should seek help from the BMA or British Dental Association (BDA) if their employment record does not allow full entitlements.

Doctors and dentists who have at least 12 months' continuous employed NHS service before the beginning of the 15th week before their expected week of confinement and plan to return to work are entitled to:

- eight weeks' full pay less Statutory Maternity Pay (SMP)
- 14 weeks' half-pay plus SMP
- four weeks' SMP
- a further 26 weeks' unpaid leave.

Doctors and dentists not intending to return to work are entitled to:

- six weeks at 9/10th of full pay
- 20 weeks at the lower rate of SMP.

Adoption leave and pay is in line with the Whitley agreement on maternity leave and pay. Doctors and dentists are eligible for full adoption pay if they have 12 months of continuous service ending with the week in which they were notified of having been matched with a child for adoption.

Under employment law doctors and dentists who are employed in the NHS are entitled to return to work under their original contract and on no less favourable terms and conditions. In addition, employers must consider requests for more flexible working arrangements. Doctors on rotations have a right to return to the same post or the next planned post, which requires careful planning by the employing trust. The doctor's original contact is extended to enable them to complete their agreed period of training.

GPs who are partners in their practice are self-employed and not covered by the Whitley agreement or statutory maternity provisions for employees. If the partnership employs a locum to cover the partner on maternity leave it will be entitled to claim a locum allowance from the PCT for up to 26 weeks, although the locum allowance is unlikely to cover the full costs of employing a locum.

Paternity and parental leave

An employee who is a mother's husband or partner is entitled to two weeks' paternity leave providing the time is being taken to support the mother or new baby, or both, and this includes same-sex partners. Doctors and dentists employed in the NHS are entitled to:

- two weeks' full pay if they have 12 months' continuous service
- two weeks' Statutory Paternity Pay if they have six months' continuous service by the 15th week before the expected date of birth.

Employees who have worked for their employer for at least 12 months can take parental leave of up to 13 weeks for each child until the child's fifth birthday.[8] Parents of disabled children born after 15 December 1994 are entitled to parental leave of 18 weeks until the child is 18 years old. Parental leave is pro rata for part-time employees. Payment during parental leave is subject to local agreement and is usually unpaid, although parental leave is regarded as continuous service.

Categories defined as continuous NHS employment for maternity, adoption, paternity, parental and sick leave

NHS employment is defined as the total periods of employment by a NHS trust, primary care trust, strategic health authority, special health authority, or any of its predecessors in England, Wales, Scotland and Northern Ireland. A break in service is disregarded for continuity of service (but not counted as a period of NHS service) when it falls into one of the following categories:

- Employment under the terms of an honorary NHS contract.
- A period of up to 12 months spent abroad as part of a definite programme of postgraduate training on the advice of the Postgraduate Dean or College or Faculty Advisor in the specialty concerned.
- A period of voluntary service overseas with a recognised international relief organisation for a period of 12 months which may, exceptionally, be extended for a further 12 months at the discretion of the employer who recruits the employee on his or her return.
- Absence on an employment break scheme in accordance with the provisions of section 6, part C of the Whitley Council Handbook.
- Absence on maternity leave (paid or unpaid) while in NHS service.

Salaried GPs should ensure their contract has a continuity clause to cover previous NHS work before joining their current practice. Model terms and conditions for salaried GPs employed by both General Medical Services (GMS) practices and primary care organisations (PCOs) were published in April 2003 as part of the supporting documentation to the new GMS contract. Continuity includes periods during which the practitioner provided primary medical services.

Other benefits

Various additional benefits are payable to employed doctors and dentists in certain circumstances. Further details can be obtained on the BMA (www.bma.org.uk) and BDA (www.bda-dentistry.org.uk) websites.

- Removal expenses may be payable, although significant discretion is left to the employer and each NHS trust has a local negotiating committee. However, a trust must reimburse removal expenses for a junior doctor or dentist who has to move to satisfy training requirements. Some deaneries have negotiated a removal expenses policy for trusts within their deanery boundaries. The tax-free limit for removal expenses is currently (2005/2006) £8000.
- Telephone: if it is a contractual requirement for the employee to have a home telephone the employer should pay for the cost of installation and rental of the telephone. Employees may also be able to negotiate the provision of a mobile phone or pager.
- Travel and subsistence allowances are payable in accordance with the *General Whitley Council Conditions of Service* when an employee is required to be away from their main place of work at the request of the employer.
- Indemnity is provided for hospital and community doctors and dentists through the NHS Indemnity Scheme. This does not cover doctors working

in general or private practice who must organise their own medical indemnity.

- Study leave makes an important contribution to the continuing professional development (CPD) of a doctor or dentist. The amount of study leave and entitlement to pay and expenses depends on the terms and conditions of employment.

Summary

The NHS provides a range of benefits for doctors and dentists, many of which are covered by the *General Whitley Council Conditions of Service.*[1] Although local alternatives can be agreed, they should be at least as favourable and most NHS employers continue to use national terms and conditions. Where disputes occur doctors and dentists are advised to use local procedures in the hope of resolving problems quickly and they should also seek advice from their relevant trade union. Independent financial advice should always be sought before changing or increasing pension investments. Doctors and dentists who have worked part-time or have portfolio careers may need specific help with their financial planning. Sadly, divorce is high among the medical profession and both parties need to ensure they have adequate financial security, including their pension arrangements.

References

1 Department of Health (2004) *General Whitley Council Conditions of Service.* Department of Health, London.

2 Gardiner M (2005) Whitley who? *BMJ Career Focus.* **June**: 235–236.

3 Department of Health (2002) *Hospital Medical and Dental Staff and Doctors and Dentists in Public Health Medicine and Community Health Services (England and Wales). Terms and Conditions of Service.* Department of Health, London.

4 NHS Pensions Agency (2004) *A Guide to the NHS Pension Scheme.* NHSP, Fleetwood.

5 Department of Health (2004) *GMS Statement of Financial Entitlements.* Department of Health, London.

6 Department of Trade and Industry (2003) *Maternity Rights.* DTI, London.

7 British Medical Association (2002) *Maternity Leave for NHS Medical Staff.* BMA, London.

8 Department of Trade and Industry (2002) *Parental Leave: a guide for employers and employees.* DTI, London.

Index